THINK AND ACT PATIENT LEARNING

This book discusses how patients learn about their illnesses and aims at supporting healthcare students and professionals to understand and respond better to the learning needs of patients.

Focusing on how patients absorb and retain health information, it promotes person-centred care in order that patients can participate more meaningfully in their treatment and care. Frequently, patients are expected to grasp a massive amount of information in a short period of time, when they may already be feeling stressed and overwhelmed, in order to participate in their care. Rather than focusing on the process of giving information, this book pays attention to how information is received, understood and acted on by the people who need it. It helps healthcare practitioners to develop the pedagogical skills they need to successfully support patients' understanding, skills and competencies to manage their self-care, health and wellbeing. Developing a new theoretical framework and an accompanying toolbox of practical strategies, it brings together the concepts of:

- Salutogenesis – keeps the reader's focus on what causes and maintains health, rather than disease.
- Sense of Coherence – which refers to how a person copes when they are ill, looking especially at ideas about comprehensibility, manageability and meaningfulness.
- Learning During Illness – describes what and how patients learn and their experiences related to theories and concepts of learning.
- Health Literacy – an ability to access, understand, appraise, and apply health information in a way that promotes health.

Offering new perspectives on how patients can be supported to cope with their illnesses and including authentic case studies, this text is an important read for nurses, doctors and allied health professionals who are concerned with patient learning, health education, health promotion, health literacy and person-centred care.

Lena Engqvist Boman, Division of Nursing, Department of Neurobiology, Care Sciences and Society, Karolinska Institutet, Sweden.

Ann Langius-Eklöf, Division of Nursing, Department of Neurobiology, Care Sciences and Society, Karolinska Institutet, Sweden.

Kay Sundberg, Division of Nursing, Department of Neurobiology, Care Sciences and Society, Karolinska Institutet, Sweden.

Josefin Wångdahl, Aging Research Center, Karolinska Institutet and Stockholm University, and Division of Nursing, Department of Neurobiology, Care Sciences and Society, Karolinska Institutet, Sweden.

THINK AND ACT PATIENT LEARNING

A Theoretical and Practical Framework

Lena Engqvist Boman, Ann Langius-Eklöf, Kay Sundberg and Josefin Wångdahl

Routledge
Taylor & Francis Group
LONDON AND NEW YORK

Designed cover image: Getty Images

First published 2027
by Routledge
4 Park Square, Milton Park, Abingdon, Oxon OX14 4RN

and by Routledge
605 Third Avenue, New York, NY 10158

Routledge is an imprint of the Taylor & Francis Group, an informa business

British Library Cataloguing-in-Publication Data
A catalogue record for this book is available from the British Library

ISBN: 978-1-032-89026-5 (hbk)
ISBN: 978-1-032-89025-8 (pbk)
ISBN: 978-1-003-54086-1 (ebk)

DOI: 10.4324/9781003540861

Typeset in times new roman
by Apex CoVantage, LLC

CONTENTS

ABOUT THE AUTHORS

Lena Engqvist Boman, Division of Nursing, Department of Neurobiology, Care Sciences and Society, Karolinska Institutet, Sweden. Lena is a registered nurse, PhD and researcher. She has worked as an educational developer and lecturer and has contributed to the development of teaching and learning at the university and in healthcare. Her research focuses on patient well-being and learning during cancer care and student learning.

Ann Langius-Eklöf, Division of Nursing, Department of Neurobiology, Care Sciences and Society, Karolinska Institutet, Sweden. She is a registered nurse, holds a PhD and is a professor of nursing. She has extensive experience of working in academia in both research and teaching. Her research is grounded on the salutogenic perspective and the concept of sense of coherence, and it is both methodological and clinical in nature.

Kay Sundberg, Division of Nursing, Department of Neurobiology, Care Sciences and Society, Karolinska Institutet, Sweden. She is a registered nurse and holds a PhD. As an associate professor, she has extensive experience in teaching and nursing research. Her research which is based on the concept of sense of coherence, focuses on person-centred care supported by digital technologies during and after cancer treatment.

Josefin Wångdahl, Aging Research Center, Karolinska Institutet and Stockholm University, and Division of Nursing, Department of Neurobiology, Care Sciences and Society, Karolinska Institutet, Sweden. She is an associate professor in public health with over ten years of experience in research on health literacy, migration and health, as well as practical public health work and health literacy education in academic and non-academic settings.

PREFACE

We, the authors of this book have taught in higher education, primarily in nursing programmes at all levels. As teachers, we are formally trained and have extensive experience in health professions education. Drawing on our clinical backgrounds in nursing and health science, we reflect on how knowledge about learning, which is well established in nursing education, is not always applied to patient learning in healthcare practice. Through academic discussions, we discovered that our clinical research perspectives were closely connected. Although our research was grounded in different theoretical foundations, we shared a focus on patient learning as a central concept across our work.

This view of learning is grounded in a constructivist paradigm, in which learners are regarded as active participants who construct understanding through individual reflection and interaction with others and the surrounding environment. This book therefore aims to encourage readers to reflect on and discuss how the content relates to their own contexts and their work with patients. Research and theory are interwoven with illustrations, reflective questions, examples, authentic cases and practical advice on how patient learning can be supported during illness.

We are grateful for the support and commitment from several people who have read the chapters, provided valuable feedback and assisted with the illustrations.

INTRODUCTION

Existing and emerging challenges in healthcare will significantly affect both healthcare professionals and patients. As healthcare develops rapidly, it is also becoming increasingly complex. With the aim of promoting optimal well-being and health in this evolving landscape, the *Think and Act Patient Learning* framework was developed. The framework builds on three theoretical perspectives: Sense of Coherence (SOC), Learning During Illness and Health Literacy. Present and future healthcare must focus on self-care for individuals living with illness or disease, or at risk of these conditions. Effective self-care, however, depends on patients being able to learn how to manage their health. Consequently, healthcare professionals must possess well-developed competencies in teaching and learning.

The World Health Organization (WHO) has recognised the importance of a holistic and person-centred approach to healthcare. Moreover a cultural shift from a traditional biomedical focus to a humanistic, person-centred approach is evident worldwide. Person-centred care prioritises the individual as a whole person rather than focusing solely on illness or disease. It emphasises respect for patients' values, preferences and needs, and actively involves them in decisions about their care. The goal is to create a partnership between healthcare professionals and patients, ensuring that care is tailored to the individual's situation. In line with this approach, the framework adopts a salutogenic perspective on health.

In this book, the patient is defined as a person with care needs related to illness, treatment and interaction with healthcare professionals. A central focus is recognising the person behind the patient in order to build a shared understanding and plan care together. The term "patient" also includes relatives and significant others who are involved in the care process. Healthcare refers to all forms of care, including primary, secondary, preventive, home-based and elderly care. Healthcare professionals refer to individuals with formal healthcare education who hold responsibility for providing and coordinating care. Healthcare staff refers to all personnel working within healthcare settings who contribute to patient care.

DOI: 10.4324/9781003540861-1

The book aims to integrate theory and practice within a new and unique framework and to clarify its meaning and significance for both healthcare professionals and patients. A strong theoretical foundation is essential in demonstrating that the framework is clinically relevant. The primary aim of the book is to show how theoretical perspectives on patient learning can inform and guide clinical practice, and to clarify its significance in patient care. The framework is intended for practical use, and the selected concepts are considered to have the potential to strengthen patient learning.

The book consists of six chapters. The first chapter provides an overview of the framework's dimensions. The following three chapters present in-depth theoretical discussions of the three concepts: SOC, Learning During Illness and Health Literacy. The fifth chapter addresses the pedagogical role of healthcare professionals, focuses on clinical applications of the pedagogical encounter and includes authentic case descriptions for practising use of the framework. Finally, the sixth chapter discusses the impact of contextual factors at the macro, meso and micro levels in implementing the framework. It highlights some prerequisites for an organisation grounded in salutogenic and person-centred perspectives and the competencies healthcare professionals need for successful implementation.

We hope that the book, in whole or in part, will serve as a valuable resource for education, competence development, clinical practice, development work and research. The framework needs to be tested in diverse ways so that it can evolve over time. Ultimately, the book is intended to benefit patients through the insights and approaches it presents.

1

THINK AND ACT PATIENT LEARNING – A FRAMEWORK

Lena Engqvist Boman, Ann Langius-Eklöf, Kay Sundberg and Josefin Wångdahl

> *Why do you think there is a need for a framework for patient learning? Reflect on what patient learning means to you. Reflect on what patient learning might mean for patients.*

People worldwide now live longer than in earlier periods, both with and without illness. The number of individuals living with long-term conditions is increasing, largely due to improved living conditions, preventive health measures and significant advances in medical diagnostics, treatment and rehabilitation. As people live longer, many live with one or multiple diseases, such as cancer, diabetes or rheumatoid arthritis. Hospital stays in secondary care are typically short and, follow-up care often relies on self-care within the context of primary care, with shorter and sometimes fragmented follow-ups that are often initiated by patients themselves. This places considerable demands on patients' knowledge, ability to cope and motivation to participate in self-care and to recognise new symptoms. It also requires healthcare professionals to have the knowledge and skills needed to support them effectively. To promote health, care must be grounded in a salutogenic perspective that prioritises patients' needs as they seek to understand and manage their situation during illness. This perspective should guide how essential health information is communicated and tailored to each patient.

Receiving information is not the same as understanding it well enough to manage one's condition or to find the motivation to follow treatment recommendations. For example, some individuals diagnosed with an illness may discontinue their medication because of side effects or for other reasons. It is important to explore how they think about their treatment and how they understand the purpose of continuing medication, namely to prevent relapse and reduce the risk of future complications. At the same time, healthcare professionals must strive to understand patients' reasons for not following recommended advice or treatment.

DOI: 10.4324/9781003540861-2

The focus of healthcare professionals needs to shift from only providing information to also ensuring that it is received and understood as intended, so that patients can learn from it and act on its content to participate in their care. This requires seeing the patient as a person who learns, rather than as a passive recipient of information. Person-centred care is recognised as a core approach for achieving high-quality care. Its philosophical foundation asserts that the person exists in relation to others, within a social context, and must be recognised and respected as such. The *Think and Act Patient Learning* framework presupposes a person-centred approach in which patients' experiences and preferences are heard and respected. A key factor is the establishment of a partnership between the healthcare professional and the patient. Patients' knowledge and understanding are prerequisites for this partnership. Furthermore, a salutogenic approach is proposed to facilitate the implementation of person-centred care. The *Think and Act Patient Learning* framework, which aims to support patients in achieving optimal health outcomes, consists of several interconnected dimensions (Figure 1.1):

- the salutogenic model of health
- sense of coherence (SOC)
- learning during illness
- health literacy
- a pedagogical encounter
- contextual factors

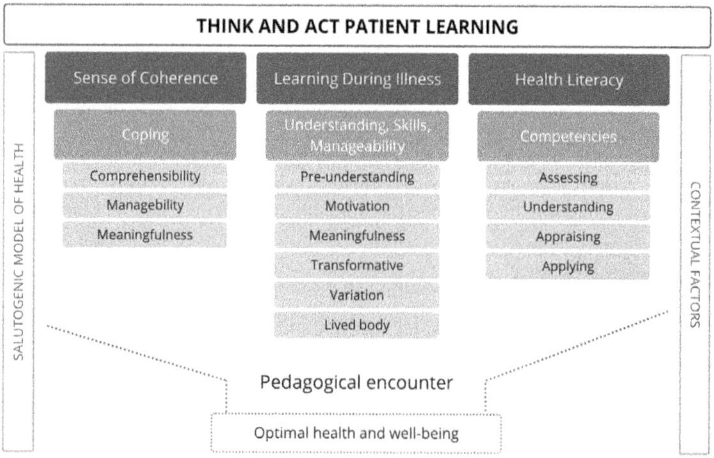

FIGURE 1.1 The *Think and Act Patient Learning* framework.

The Salutogenic Model of Health

Across the healthcare system, health should remain the central focus, reflected in governing documents, professional work and everyday patient interactions. Health is a multifaceted concept that has evolved over time and carries different meanings depending on the context. The foundation of the *Think and Act Patient Learning* framework is grounded in the salutogenic model of health, which is guided by the central question "what makes people healthy?" in contrast to the more traditional pathogenic approach that focuses on the causes of illness. Rooted in theories of stress and coping, the salutogenic model emphasises health-promoting factors within the individual that enable them to manage life challenges effectively.

Aaron Antonovsky coined the salutogenic orientation to health, challenging the traditional divide between "healthy" and "sick" and describing health as a continuum from ease to dis-ease. To cite Antonovsky, "we all are, as long as there is a breath of life in us, to some measure healthy" (Antonovsky, 1987). Salutogenesis focuses on aspects that actively promote health by using a person's own resources. From this perspective, health does not necessarily imply the absence of disease but includes the person's subjective experience and perception of health in relation to illness and disease. It conceptualises health as a dynamic process, focusing on promoting and maintaining well-being and quality of life. The emphasis is on the interaction between individuals and their environment, as well as on personal resources. A salutogenic view of health also provides an explicit perspective on individual processes during a ease and disease trajectory. Central to this are patients' individual needs and preferences, integrated with healthcare professionals' competence.

The overarching aim of patient learning is for the patient to acknowledge and strengthen their own capacity for self-care in order to reach optimal health and well-being. Patient learning, therefore, requires a holistic view of the individual, focusing not only on disease but also on personal preferences, resources and social context. The patient should be an active participant and valued partner in the care team, rather than a passive recipient.

> *A salutogenic approach to patient learning focuses on patients' understanding of their illness and on strengthening the resources that enable confidence, capability and active participation in care and health promotion.*

Think and Act Patient Learning – Three Theoretical Perspectives

The framework shows how patient learning can be understood from three theoretical perspectives: SOC, learning during illness and health literacy. These perspectives are grounded in research on individuals' overall coping capacity, how people learn while living with illness and how their information skills shape this process. Together, they are clinically relevant for developing in-depth knowledge and serve as key foundations for understanding patient learning. SOC describes a patient's overall capacity to cope with stressors and influences how patients interpret their situation and their capability to engage in learning during illness. The concept reflects an individual's ability to comprehend, manage and find meaning in stressful situations, such as living with or being at risk of disease. Learning during illness focuses on the patient's learning process as they adapt to a changed life situation. It involves developing understanding, skills and strategies to manage the challenges associated with illness. Health literacy concerns an individual's ability to access, understand, appraise and apply health information in ways that offer a practical and actionable path for improving health outcomes. The three perspectives are interconnected, as all learning processes involve engaging with information to make sense of the world and to manage various situations effectively.

The individual's motivation and ability to obtain information and interact with the environment are fundamental for how learning progresses (Illeris, 2009). Learning during illness shares many aspects with learning in general but is distinguished by the expectation that the patient will learn, often in a threatening situation that may involve strong emotions (Engqvist Boman et al., 2017). Important aspects of learning include the patient's pre-understanding, motivation and experience of meaningfulness, transformation and variation through the lived body during illness. Pre-understanding refers to the individual's knowledge, perceptions, thoughts and experiences, which influence the learning process. Motivational factors for learning during illness are intrusive and deeply personal, as the illness affects the individual's body, mind and overall life situation. A key driving force for learning is meaningfulness, that is, when the learner perceives the information as relevant, understands it and can apply it. Pre-understanding plays a crucial role in this meaning-making process because new information is interpreted in relation to it. For some, the experience of having an illness contributes to transformative learning with a changed understanding of themselves and their outlook on life. Learning is triggered by variation, that is, the experience that something is different and captured by the individual's awareness. Patients' awareness of variation in their bodies or changes in the environment can be important sources of information. Patients collect information through the lived body with all senses activated, and their bodily signals are continuously interpreted in relation to their pre-understanding. Patients need to express their interpretation of information and experiences to receive feedback on their understanding, skills and manageability.

For patients to take an active role in advice, treatment and self-care, they must develop an understanding of, and an ability to handle, their changed health circumstances. SOC reflects an individual's overall capacity to do so, including the extent to which they are motivated to engage in these activities. This underscores the importance of considering and addressing health literacy in clinical and educational settings, as it can enhance patients' ability to access, understand, appraise and apply health information (Sørensen et al., 2021). These competencies are essential for navigating healthcare systems, making informed health decisions and engaging in health-promoting activities and self-care. Research clearly demonstrates that an individual's ability to manage and adapt to illness has a direct impact on the course of their healthcare and health trajectory. An individual's degree of SOC is essential for how they cope with illness and is considered a personality characteristic (Antonovsky, 1987). Those with a higher degree of SOC adapt to illness and perceive better health and well-being than those with lower degrees. The degree of SOC also underpins the choice, conscious or unconscious, of different coping strategies. Individuals with a high SOC tend to employ a broad repertoire of coping strategies, adapted to the nature of the stressor, whether it is a daily hassle, a major life event or a chronic condition. Consequently, healthcare professionals must recognise that each patient possesses a unique pattern of coping strategies, has varying degrees of SOC and health literacy, and must be supported accordingly. This also applies to patients' different ways of learning and how they understand their situation. Moreover, healthcare professionals often place patients in situations they are expected to cope with. These include receiving information about test results, medical procedures, preparing for surgery, screening or learning to manage a diagnosis such as diabetes or high blood pressure. At the same time, healthcare professionals should consider the patient's degree of SOC and health literacy and support them in accessing, understanding, appraising and applying health information. This includes removing barriers such as unclear or inaccessible information and helping patients navigate the healthcare system in a way that fits their cognitive and physical abilities as well as their pre-understanding. This is important, as health literacy is linked to many health outcomes, including health behaviours, use of healthcare services and overall health status. Individuals with a low SOC and limited health literacy often face additional challenges, which may be linked to lower educational attainment and socio-economic status. These factors can increase their vulnerability to a poorer quality of life, reduced well-being and even higher risks of morbidity and mortality. To think and act in a learning-oriented way therefore means supporting the patient's learning process during illness, as well as strengthening their coping abilities and health literacy. At the same time, those who are less vulnerable, due to their access to health-promoting resources, also need attention to ensure that they can navigate the healthcare landscape successfully and receive sufficient support throughout their learning process.

An individual's abilities and resources to manage stressful situations are prerequisites for their well-being and optimal health. These abilities include effectively engaging with relevant information in ways that support understanding and informed action. As with all learning, the individual needs time to process information, which involves taking in and interacting with the content and with others, such as healthcare professionals, family and friends. In this interaction, feedback from experts is crucial to minimise lack of understanding or misunderstanding. In healthcare encounters, it is essential to identify health-promoting factors and explore how each situation can be made comprehensible, manageable and meaningful for the patient. Together, these elements shape how individuals respond to stressors such as illness or the threat of illness, influencing the overall health trajectory, including the transition from being healthy to becoming a patient. More recently, health literacy has been proposed as a key resource within the salutogenic model, supporting individuals as they navigate transitions from disorder to order (Saboga-Nunes et al., 2019). Transformative learning may occur when a challenging or disruptive event triggers a deep, structural shift in how individuals understand themselves, their relationships and their world (Mezirow, 2009). This process goes beyond acquiring new information and can lead to major changes in personal values and in how individuals prioritise their time, lifestyle and relationships. SOC, learning during illness, and health literacy are key perspectives in supporting patient learning. A salutogenic approach to patient encounters enhances healthcare professionals' understanding of how patients learn and promotes improved health and well-being.

> *Conceptual knowledge of SOC, learning during illness and health literacy is important for understanding how patients learn which is crucial for supporting them achieving optimal health and well-being.*

Pedagogical Encounter

A pedagogical encounter is a learning situation where the learner interacts with someone or something to develop their understanding, manageability and skills. Thinking and acting from a patient learning perspective means that healthcare professionals base their actions on knowledge of how patients learn within the pedagogical encounter. Pedagogical encounters can involve both planned and unplanned learning situations or organised patient education provided over a shorter or longer period, either individually or in a group, such as:

- consultation with a doctor about diagnosis and treatment
- practicing with a nurse how to perform self-care of a wound
- rehabilitation exercises after hip fracture with the support of a physiotherapist
- using assistive devices at home together with an occupational therapist
- discussion with a dietitian about healthy eating
- telephone consultation with healthcare professionals
- a spontaneous meeting in connection with a visit to the hospital
- group education for patients after their heart attack

The model of pedagogical encounter presented by Silén (2013), includes the use of theories about learning. A pedagogical encounter is always related to a situation, which affects the learning. A planned pedagogical encounter includes a structure with three phases (before, during and after the encounter) and eight aspects: the situation, agents, purpose, goals, intentions, interaction, content, and learning activities (Figure 1.2). The agents involved can be students, teachers, patients, healthcare professionals or others. Purpose, goals,

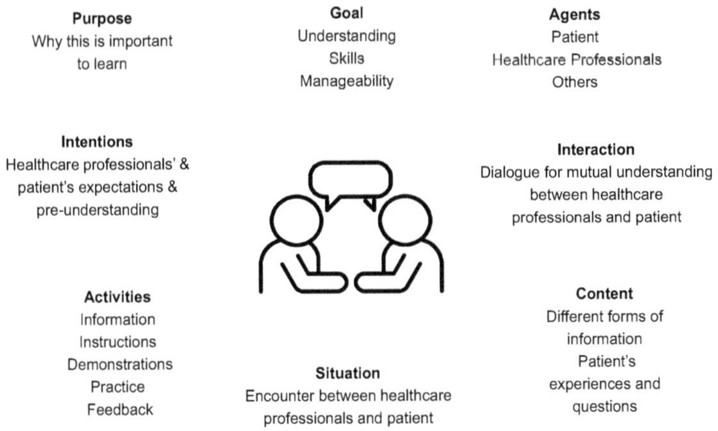

FIGURE 1.2 Pedagogical encounter.

Illustration created with Canva and adapted from Silén (2013, p. 27)

content and activities need to be clarified, as well as the patient's and healthcare professionals' intentions for the encounter. All agents in a pedagogical encounter can interact and learn from each other; that is, a patient learns from experts in healthcare and the experts learn from the patient.

The aspects of a pedagogical encounter are exemplified in a meeting between a nurse and a patient with prostate cancer (Box 1.1).

BOX 1.1 EXAMPLE OF A PEDAGOGICAL ENCOUNTER

Situation

A preoperative meeting between a patient recently diagnosed with prostate cancer and a nurse takes place in a room in an outpatient surgery department at a university hospital.

Agents

The patient, their partner, a nurse, a nursing student and a medical student participate in the meeting.

Purpose

To follow up on the patient's feelings and understanding of the situation, and to inform and prepare the patient for surgical treatment of prostate cancer.

Goals

At the end of the encounter, the patient understands what will happen, what he needs to do to prepare for the surgery, how he may feel post-operatively and what he needs to do after returning home. He knows how to perform the subcutaneous injection and understands that it prevents thrombosis. The patient and his partner have received answers to their questions and concerns and know who to contact after discharge from the hospital.

Intentions

The nurse's intention is to make the patient feel safe and ensure that he understands what will happen. The nurse asks the patient how he is feeling and what his expectations are for the meeting.

Interaction

The patient's and partner's thoughts and questions initiate and guide the encounter. The nurse creates a dialogue, asks open-ended questions and continuously checks their understanding after information and instructions have been given.

Content

Written and verbal information on preoperative preparations, along with instructions supported by visual aids and demonstrations on how to perform a subcutaneous injection. The content is adapted to the patient's and partner's pre-understanding, concerns and questions related to the treatment and care of the patient's illness.

Learning Activities

The nurse provides information, instructions and demonstrations and ensures – by letting the patient teach-back – that the information is understandable, manageable and used as intended. The patient practices how to perform the injection and receives feedback from the nurse.

Think and Act Patient Learning from a Salutogenic Perspective

Healthcare professionals need to apply a salutogenic and person-centred approach, supported by theoretical knowledge of SOC, learning during illness and health literacy. They need to draw on this knowledge to think and act from a patient-learning perspective in both planned and unplanned learning situations involving patients and their relatives. In such encounters, adopting a salutogenic perspective means focusing on the patient's needs and the resources they have available. This is achieved by creating a dialogue aimed at mutual understanding, assessing patients' and relatives' needs, pre-understanding and resources, and providing accessible health information. A pedagogical encounter involves supporting patients in navigating the healthcare system. The three theoretical perspectives on patient learning within the framework overlap to some extent, and the aspects in common provide a basis for thinking and acting patient learning. These include patient's pre-understanding, sense of meaningfulness and motivation to learn, perceptions through the lived body, ability to process information and experiences, understanding, manageability, skills and competencies, and health-promoting resources. Pre-understanding encompasses the individual's knowledge, experiences, health beliefs and attitudes that can influence their understanding and manageability of the current situation and information. Meaningfulness means that the content must be relevant and understandable. Motivation is related to meaningfulness and is important in all learning, but patients also experience both external and internal drives to learn. Learning through the lived body is an ongoing process during illness and includes variation in experiences and interpretations of stimuli from the senses and emotions. Processing all kinds of information and experiences is necessary to construct one's understanding through, for example, reading, thinking, talking to others, practising and receiving feedback.

The purpose of creating a salutogenic pedagogical encounter within healthcare is to support the patient's health and well-being during illness (Figure 1.3). The overall goal is that patients understand their situation and can make informed decisions about their health and well-being. To support this, an allowing atmosphere should be ensured to promote mutual understanding, where the patient feels seen and respected. When these conditions are in place, patients are more likely to make sound judgements, cope with their illness and strengthen their health and well-being.

The common aspects of thinking and acting in patient learning need to be considered in all pedagogical encounters with patients. Planning, performing and evaluating such encounters is often possible during longer meetings that

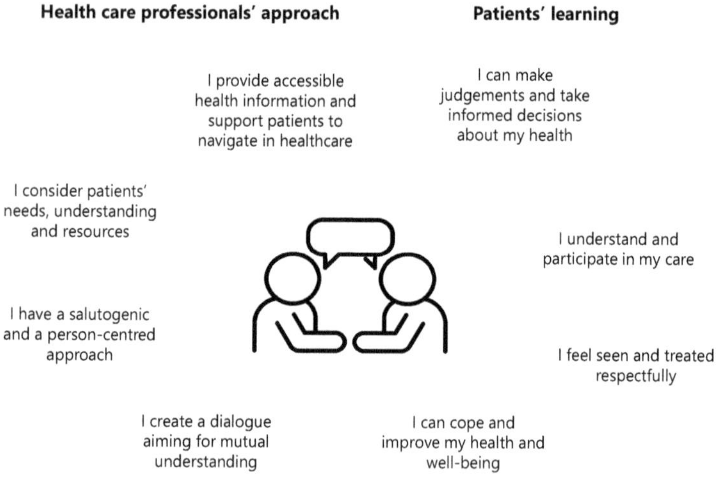

FIGURE 1.3 Salutogenic pedagogical encounter.

Illustration created with Canva.

involve patients, their relatives and healthcare professionals. However, most interactions in healthcare are brief and cannot always be thoroughly planned, for example, in acute situations, in digital health settings or when time is limited. In all of these circumstances, healthcare professionals' knowledge and competence in thinking and acting patient learning become crucial and must be applied with great flexibility and sensitivity, as described in greater detail in the following chapters.

Contextual Factors

Contextual factors such as societal and organisational structures and resources influence the implementation of the *Think and Act Patient Learning* framework in healthcare. Implementation of interventions is dependent on contexts at the macro, meso and micro levels in healthcare organisations (Fulop & Robert, 2015). The macro level involves the national policy context, while the meso level encompasses the organisational context, including leadership, culture and systems. The micro level corresponds to the units where the framework is implemented and concerns stakeholders such as patients, students and healthcare professionals. It can be difficult for healthcare professionals to influence the organisation of healthcare at a macro level. At the meso level, a healthcare organisation, such as a hospital, may decide to implement person-centred care. This, in turn, may support healthcare development at a micro level, such as an outpatient clinic or care unit. To implement the *Think and Act Patient Learning* framework, healthcare professionals need to learn how to support patients in relation to their SOC, learning process and health literacy in pedagogical encounters. The healthcare organisation and its management need to organise and follow up on such competence development.

Summary

The *Think and Act Patient Learning* framework offers perspectives on patient learning anchored in a salutogenic approach to health and in individuals' health-promoting resources. A patient's resources can be strengthened by supporting their SOC, learning during illness and health literacy. Central to the framework is meeting patients' needs in pedagogical encounters by thinking and acting from a patient learning perspective. Salutogenic pedagogical encounters are characterised by mutual understanding and by the patient feeling seen, heard and respected. The goal is to enable patients to understand their health situation and make informed decisions that support optimal health outcomes. In the subsequent Chapters 2, 3 and 4, the theoretical perspectives on patient learning – SOC, learning during illness and health literacy – are discussed in greater depth. Chapter 5 provides guidance on how healthcare professionals can create pedagogical encounters by thinking and acting from a patient learning perspective. Chapter 6 addresses how contextual factors influence the implementation of the *Think and Act Patient Learning* framework within an organisation.

References

Antonovsky, A. (1987). *Unraveling the mystery of health: How people manage stress and stay well.* Jossey-Bass.

Engqvist Boman, L., Sandelin, K., Wengström, Y., & Silén, C. (2017). Patients' learning and understanding during their breast cancer trajectory. *Patient Education and Counselling*, 100, 795–804. https://doi.org/10.1016/j.pec.2016.12.024

Fulop, N., & Robert, G. (2015). *Context for successful quality improvement.* The Health Foundation.

Illeris, K. (2009). *Contemporary theories of learning: Learning theorists . . . in their own words.* Routledge.

Mezirow, J. (2009). An overview on transformative learning. In K. Illeris (Ed.), *Contemporary theories of learning: Learning theorists . . . in their own words* (pp. 90–105). Routledge.

Saboga-Nunes, L., Bittlingmayer, U., & Okan, O. (2019). Salutogenesis and health literacy: The health promotion simplex! In O. Okan, U. Bauer, D. Levin-Zamir, P. Pinheiro, & K. Sørensen (Eds.), *International handbook of health literacy: Research, practice and policy across the life span.* Policy Press. https://doi.org/10.51952/9781447344520.ch042

Silén, C. (2013). Learning in the medicine and health care field [Lärande inom medicin och vårdområdet]. In C. Silén & K. Bolander Laksov (Eds.), *Creating pedagogical encounters in medicine and health care* [Att skapa pedagogiska möten i medicin och vård]. Studentlitteratur.

Sørensen, K., Levin-Zamir, D., Duong, T. V., Okan, O., Brasil, V. V., & Nutbeam, D. (2021). Building health literacy system capacity: A framework for health literate systems. *Health Promotion International*, 36(Suppl. 1), i13–i23. https://doi.org/10.1093/heapro/daab153

2

SALUTOGENESIS AND SENSE OF COHERENCE

Ann Langius-Eklöf and Kay Sundberg

Can you think of a situation where you met someone and were surprised at how they managed to cope with a considerably stressful situation? Reflect on what you believe helped that person handle the situation.

In this chapter, the salutogenic model of health and the concept of sense of coherence (SOC) are described. The model of salutogenesis, coined by Aaron Antonovsky in 1979, has been extensively acknowledged globally. The focus in the model is on how health can be strengthened, promoted and preserved in patients who have or live at risk of disease or illness. The concept of SOC aims to explain why some people cope better with strain than others. Patients' own experiences and preferences in relation to a disease, or a threatened medical condition, are fundamental in how they can learn to be involved in their demanding situation. The chapter includes descriptions and theoretical assumptions of the model of salutogenesis and the concept of SOC. They have been applied in several disciplines, mostly within public science and healthcare science. In this chapter, the focus is from a healthcare perspective.

Health and Well-Being

The concept of health has several meanings depending on the context and has been developed over time. Perspectives that have been influential are mainly philosophical, biomedical, sociological, psychological, political and ethical. In the healthcare sector, health is a central concept at many levels, from governing documents and policies to health professions and patients. In this sector, there are two main views on health: the biomedical and the humanistic perspectives. The biomedical perspective has been dominant since the 16th century, when Vesalius produced detailed mappings of the human body's anatomy, which led to rapid development of medicine, particularly in surgical practice. This development was reinforced by the assumption that body and soul are separate entities, which established the unique status of the biomedical perspective,

DOI: 10.4324/9781003540861-3

defining health primarily as the absence of disease. Influences from philosophical, sociological and psychological perspectives have subsequently emphasised that the human being is a unified entity of body and soul. In 1946, WHO's definition of health was expanded to "Health is a state of complete physical, mental and social well-being and not merely the absence of disease or infirmity" which is a fundamental human right (World Health Organization, 1946), a statement with a clear paradigm shift from the view that the definition of health originated solely from the biomedical perspective.

Health being more than the absence of disease also meant not seeing health as static but rather as a dynamic process, something individuals perceive in their daily life, often in relation to a disease or at risk for disease. This was illustrated in a Health Cross model by Katie Eriksson (Eriksson, 1984), a philosopher in caring science. The model enables theoretical and practical understanding, integrating the humanistic and biomedical perspectives in healthcare (Figure 2.1).

The WHO health definition from 1946 has mainly been criticised for being overly idealistic and broad. In recent decades, however, the health paradigm has evolved to incorporate more nuanced perspectives, addressing health at

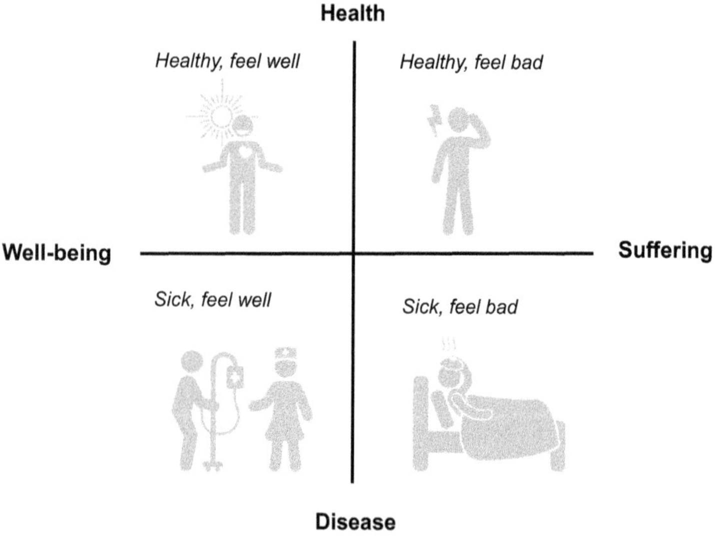

FIGURE 2.1 Illustration of the integration of the humanistic and biomedical perspectives on health according to Eriksson's Health Cross.

Illustration created with Canva.

the individual, group and societal levels. Moreover, health risks and consequences of, for instance, smoking, unhealthy food, poverty, war, natural disasters and unemployment are important to prevent. Although the original definition remains unchanged, the growing focus on health promotion has reframed health as a resource for everyday life and as a positive concept that emphasises not only physical capabilities but also social and personal assets (World Health Organization, 1986). A key semantic criticism of the WHO definition is its utopian portrayal of health as "a state of complete physical, mental, and social well-being" which implies that, by this standard, most people are almost always considered unhealthy. This critique was a major factor leading Antonovsky to develop the salutogenic model of health.

The Salutogenic Model of Health

Aaron Antonovsky (1923–1994) was a medical sociologist whose research fields spanned cancer, multiple sclerosis and cardiovascular diseases. He discovered that he was more interested in the psychosocial aspects than the diseases per se. Through research in the late 1970s, he further conceptualised health to what he called "The Salutogenic Model of Health" (Antonovsky, 1979).

Salutogenesis means the origin of health and is the opposite of pathogenesis (the origin of disease). From the salutogenic perspective, health is a dynamic process that changes during life and sometimes from day to day. Antonovsky visualised this on a continuum with two opposite extremes: absolute dis-ease and absolute ease (Figure 2.2). The continuum represents the balance between the opposite poles, indicating that an individual will be positioned somewhere along the spectrum throughout life. Regardless of where an individual is situated on this continuum, they always possess some degree of health, which serves as an essential resource for daily life.

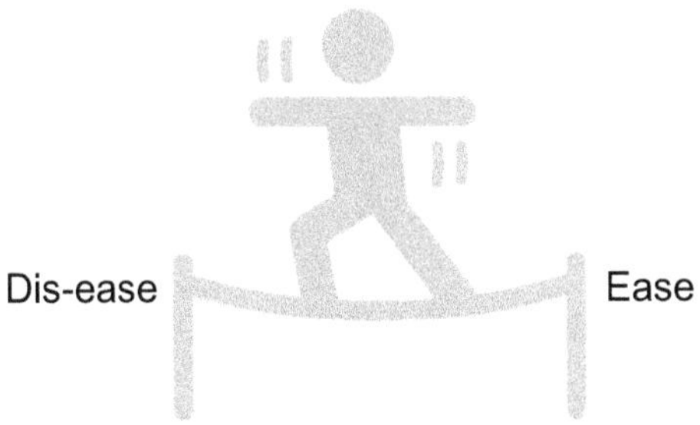

FIGURE 2.2 The health continuum.

Illustration created with Canva

Central to the salutogenic model is the interaction between people, not only what is ongoing within the individual. The construction of society and the resources and structure in an individual's own life are considered equally important. The main questions in the salutogenic model are "Why do people have health?" and "How do people manage to stay healthy?" This way of viewing health is very different to the pathogenic perspective, where the individual is assessed by either being sick or well, an organ being sick or well, a condition being pathological or not, or whether the presence of risk factors for disease exists or not.

In a pathogenic approach, success is evaluated primarily based on improvement of disease or increased life expectancy. It is self-evident that diseases can be prevented or cured and/or alleviated. Within the salutogenic perspective, success is evaluated through indicators such as enhanced well-being or subjective health, increased self-care capacity and the individual's ability to adapt to disease. The salutogenic perspective focuses on health and well-being and originates from identifying health-promoting factors, opportunities and success factors rather than problems, risk factors and obstacles. However, in healthcare, the salutogenic perspective and the pathogenic perspective should not be seen as opposites but rather as a complement to each other (Figure 2.3). In other words, these perspectives are not mutually exclusive, as both perspectives are interplayed to achieve evidence-based healthcare. For example, education for physicians focuses on the pathogenic perspective and for nurses the salutogenic, but both professions have insight into each other's perspectives.

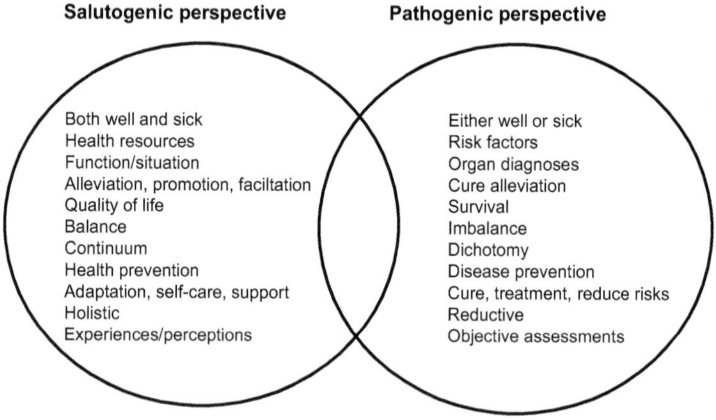

FIGURE 2.3 Illustration of the balance between the salutogenic and pathogenic perspectives.

TABLE 2.1 Health and care needs differ between individuals and situations

X with broken arm. *Just fix it*	Concrete needs related to disease.	X newly diagnosed with diabetes. *"Give me all information to handle this".*	Concrete needs related to disease.
Y with broken arm. *I need help to manage my work as I am dependent of my arm*	Needs in relation to body and soul.	Y newly diagnosed with diabetes. *I need support to take blood sugar tests; I am afraid of infections.*	Needs in relation to body and soul.
Z with broken arm. *How can I be a good parent? I am a single mom of three small kids and they need food, clothes and a pain-free mom.*	Existential needs, related to life goals.	X newly diagnosed with diabetes. *Am I going to die now? What about my family?*	Existential needs, related to life goals.

It should be noted that individuals' subjective values of their own health, quality of life and well-being are not always congruent with professionals' assessment of the individuals' values. Furthermore, just as an objective state (having a disease or a risk factor) can predict how an individual rates well-being, subjective ratings can predict both mortality and morbidity (Haring et al., 2011; Sajjad et al., 2017). When meeting patients, it is important to reflect on the individual's own healthcare needs, which should be considered in combination with professional competence (Table 2.1).

What was innovative in Antonovsky's reasoning was that, unlike previous approaches, he fundamentally theorised what contributes to the origin of health – an area that had not been systematically explored before. One of the most important resources in the salutogenic model is the individual's overall view and approach to their own life and context, defined by the concept of SOC, which in turn affects how an individual can handle various events in life such as being affected by disease or illness.

The Concept of SOC

SOC, as the central concept in the salutogenic model by Aaron Antonovsky, reflects an individual's view of life and resources to maintain health, especially during times of considerable strain (Antonovsky, 1987). Antonovsky defined SOC as a person's global orientation in life and the extent to which a person sees the world as ordered, making sense and possible to be handled. The concept of SOC aims to explain why some people adapt more successfully to considerable strain than others and thereby move towards the healthy pole (ease) on the continuum. Hence, a crucial factor for the direction an individual moves towards on the continuum is their degree of SOC in life. A high SOC is dependent on the individual's confidence that: (i) the stimuli from one's internal and external environments in life are structured, predictable and explicable; (ii) the resources are available to meet the demands posed by these stimuli; and (iii) these demands are challenges, worthy of investment and engagement. These dimensions are described by the three components of comprehensibility, manageability and meaningfulness.

- Comprehensibility is a cognitive dimension that reflects the extent to which an individual perceives events (a problem or a current issue) as making sense, either those occurring in their environment or affecting them personally. It involves viewing the world as rational, structured and ordered rather than unclear and chaotic. The extremes are order and chaos, structure and randomness, and coherence and inexplicability.
- Manageability reflects the extent of the belief of understanding the problem and having the necessary resources at disposal to handle the problem successfully. These resources can be perceived as sufficient or as being controlled by others or fate. Available resources can be within the individual or in the environment, such as relatives, healthcare staff and friends. The extremes are a feeling of always being able to handle situations or the experience that it is only depending on others or something else, for example, rules.
- Meaningfulness is the motivational dimension and considered to be the most important component, reflecting the extent to which an individual feels engaged and that handling the situation is worthwhile and makes sense. Meaningfulness represents an individual's perception of motivation in life and that life has emotional meaning. In this component, a feeling of being engaged and seeing challenges is one extreme, and the other is the absence of the feeling that there is something of importance in life.

These three components are typically intertwined, meaning that individuals often experience all three simultaneously to various degrees (Figure 2.4). Experiencing low meaningfulness and at the same time high comprehensibility and manageability seems as unlikely as low comprehensibility and meaningfulness providing high manageability. Having the ability to handle stressful situations presupposes in most cases that an individual understands and sees structure in life events and feels motivated to be able to influence. On the other hand, if there is a high sense of meaningfulness, there may be a possibility that it compensates for low comprehensibility and manageability.

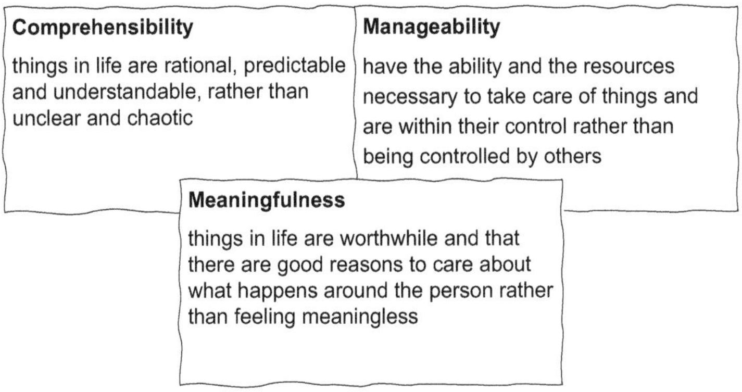

FIGURE 2.4 The three components of SOC – comprehensibility, manageability and meaningfulness – are intertwined.

The theoretical assumption is that how successfully stressful situations are handled depends on an individual's level of SOC in life. A high SOC is assumed to contribute to successful management and thus to better health and quality of life. The corresponding assumption for low SOC is that it contributes to less successful coping and thus to poorer health and quality of life (Figure 2.5).

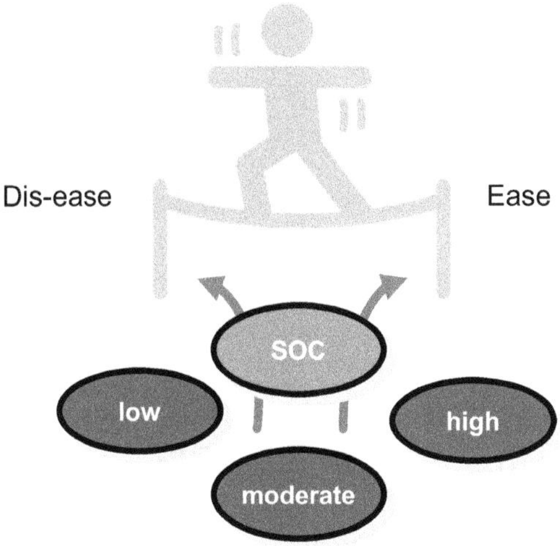

FIGURE 2.5 The degree of SOC in relation to position on the health continuum.

Illustration created with Canva.

The Development of SOC

In Antonovsky's theoretical reasoning, the individual's basic SOC develops from infancy to early adulthood (Antonovsky, 1987; Mittelmark et al., 2017). The development of SOC during childhood, adolescence and early adulthood is multifactorial. Important factors are childhood experiences and social, cultural and historical contexts. In the salutogenic model, Antonovsky discusses various health-promoting factors, which he called General Resistance Resources, that an individual has at their disposal from early life. These are individual factors such as preventive approach, economic and material standard, education, self-identity, social support, beliefs, cultural stability and genetic factors (Table 2.2).

Antonovsky leant towards scientific evidence for his assumptions that the general resistance resources are important for health and thereby crucial for an individual's successful stress management and the development of the degree of SOC. Numerous research has shown that those with good living conditions and a good education have a greater chance of staying healthy and moving towards the healthy side of the continuum. Having good self-awareness is also a factor that is considered to have a positive effect on health. It is well-known that social support is an important buffer against disease and illness. Being committed to what you do, feeling cultural stability and having a compelling belief in something (not necessarily a religious belief) also have a positive effect on health. An individual's preventive approach and genetic predisposition are also of great importance for the development of SOC. Recently, health literacy has been suggested as an addition to Antonovsky's list of generalised resistance resources (Saboga-Nunes et al., 2019). The degree of SOC achieved in adulthood depends on the balance between how different life experiences are understood and managed and how meaningful this has appeared in early years. The role of the general resistance resources for development of SOC is evident, and having a high SOC helps the individual to identify and mobilise the resistance resources to handle stressors and manage tension successfully.

TABLE 2.2 General resistance resources important in the development of an individual's SOC

Material	Cultural stability
Knowledge	Magic
Ego identity	Religion/philosophy
Coping strategies	Preventive approach
Social support	Health literacy
Commitment	Genetic factors

The SOC Scale

Antonovsky not only defined the concept of SOC as the basis of the salutogenic perspective but also developed an instrument (the SOC scale) to be able to measure and scientifically test the concept (Antonovsky, 1987; Mittelmark et al., 2017). He wanted to confirm his assumption that those with higher SOC deal with stressful situations in a more successful way and thus have better health and quality of life.

The development of the SOC scale was scientifically extensive. The first phase consisted of 51 in-depth interviews with people who had undergone severe life crises such as loss of loved ones, imprisonment in concentration camps or serious disabilities. The interviews formed the basis for a faceted classification design used to develop the scale. This is a specific sociological method that is used mainly when global and dynamic concepts are to be described. Based on the interviews and with the help of the facets, Antonovsky formulated several items that were assumed to reflect the concept of SOC. He then systematically processed and tested the statements until finally 29 items remained that made up the SOC scale. A shorter, 13-item version of the scale is also available and has been more commonly used in nursing research. The systematic procedure for developing the SOC scale means that if the original content of the questions changes, there is a risk that the concept of SOC is lost.

It is suggested in the distribution of the SOC value in the population that a quarter have low or high SOC, and half a moderate one. Furthermore, a clinically significant change in the SOC score is suggested if the change occurs between these three boundaries. The instrument has been translated into over 50 languages and has shown good measurement properties in terms of both reliability and validity (Eriksson & Mittelmark, 2017). Several studies moreover show that when using the SOC scale for group comparisons, the short version is as reliable and valid as the long version.

The Stability of SOC

In young adults, SOC can fluctuate, but by the time the individual reaches the age of 30, SOC is assumed to be relatively stable. Antonovsky hypothesised that the degree of SOC in young adulthood is deeply rooted and that the degree of SOC can only temporarily change when important and/or extremely stressful events occur in life. For example, disease diagnosis can lead to a crisis, making life seem more incomprehensible, unmanageable and meaningless than usual. On the other hand, if a major positive event occurs, life will likely become more comprehensible, manageable and meaningful at that moment. Antonovsky assumed that in such situations, the degree of SOC will eventually return to its original degree when the temporary event is over.

The stability of SOC has been shown in numerous studies, although an increase over time has been seen in some populations (Sundberg et al., 2022). There have been a few intervention studies with the intent of improving SOC through, for example, rehabilitation and patient education programmes or structured nursing support for strengthening coping and self-care. However, the clinical effects were small and the follow-up periods relatively short, and more evidence is needed to conclude whether any stable improvement in SOC remains.

SOC and Coping Strategies

Stress is commonly defined as the state of tension that an individual experiences when faced with a demand that the individual must manage in some way (Lazarus & Folkman, 1984). Stress research is commonly focused on studying the nature of the stimulus, the individual's handling and choice of strategies, and the context in which it arises. Each stimulus encountered is cognitively assessed as either irrelevant, neutral or threatening. This process is termed coping, and the specific ways an individual handles a stimulus are termed coping strategies. Stimuli that can affect humans can be divided into three different types. Chronic stimuli are those that are essentially beyond the control of the individual, such as natural disasters, war or famine. Life events are stimuli that affect the individual, involving one or a few people in their vicinity, such as the death of a close relative, illness, divorce or childbirth. The third form of stimulus is daily hassles, such as missing the bus, giving a lecture, feeling lonely, undergoing an X-ray, waiting for rounds or having a dispute with somebody. Antonovsky emphasises, more clearly than other theorists, that stimuli capable of causing stressful situations can also be positive and necessary. For some, stress can even be a spice of life. Understanding how humans are constantly exposed to and handling stimuli, even seemingly less demanding ones, is extremely important for healthcare professionals. It is worth considering that for some patients, situations such as having to wait a long time for a physician examination or sharing a room with another patient can be much more stressful than for others and can have negative consequences.

Most of the research aimed at studying stress management has focused on investigating which strategies contribute to poorer or better management and thus to poorer health and quality of life. There are a variety of strategies described in the literature that humans use to varying degrees to cope with strain (Table 2.3). Antonovsky meant that the individual's pattern and flexibility in using different strategies is probably more interesting than seeking knowledge of which strategies are better or worse (Antonovsky, 1987). He emphasised that SOC is not a coping strategy, but rather a prerequisite for the choices of strategies that the individual makes. There have been some studies on a

TABLE 2.3 Coping strategies

Anxiety/exercise	Accept situation
Discuss problem	Withdraw from situation
View problem objectively	Worry
Maintain control	Eat/smoke/use drugs
Find purpose/meaning	Daydream
Try to change situation	Get mad
Seek comfort/help from others	Get nervous
Try out solutions	Blame others for problem
Make use of past experiences	Take tension out of others
Handle problem in steps	Except the worst
Set goals	Want to be alone
Information-seeking	Self-pity
Seeks social support	Cry
Put problem aside	Optimism
Let others solve problem	Pessimism
Try anything	Fighting spirit
Pray	Helplessness
Resignation because it is hopeless	Denial
Sleep	Wishful thinking
Don't worry	Avoidance
Compromise	Isolation
Do nothing and wait it out	Self-control
Hope for improvement	Shared concern
Laugh if off	Confrontation
Resignation because it is fate	Fatalism
Humour	Distancing

person's SOC and choice of strategies to handle a specific stressful situation, showing strikingly similar patterns in healthy and sick people.

SOC and Adaptation to Stressful Situations or Disease

The theoretical assumption that an individual's ability to cope with considerable strain or disease depends on a person's degree of SOC is also scientifically evident. The SOC scale has frequently been used in healthcare research to explore how SOC relates to various outcomes of individuals' experience in connection with a disease (Sundberg et al., 2022). Research consistently shows that a higher SOC helps to mobilise an individual's resources to manage tension successfully, contributing to better health and well-being. Higher SOC relates to patients' perceptions of higher psychological and psychosocial well-being and quality of life irrespective of their medical condition. Moreover, individuals with a low SOC tend to have more serious consequences from disease and a higher risk for poorer health and health-related quality of life. Some studies indicate that SOC negatively relates to comorbidity and even death. For example, women diagnosed with breast cancer who had a low SOC at the time of diagnosis showed a substantially increased risk of disease progression and breast cancer-related death as well as all-cause mortality ten years later (Lindblad et al., 2018). This link between low SOC and increased mortality may coincide with failure to adhere to long-term hormonal therapy. It was hypothesised that in relation to the severe side effects of treatment, patients with low SOC might not fully understand the importance of taking the medication and thereby not be motivated to do so. There are also studies showing that the degree of SOC can be associated with objective health measures (Sundberg et al., 2022). Some results point to high SOC relating to shorter sick leave, lower blood sugar, lower blood pressure and better adherence to treatment. The role of SOC in a life-threatening situation was studied during the Covid-19 pandemic, and results showed that SOC was an important personal resource for dealing with fear (Dymecka et al., 2021). Numerous studies show that SOC can serve as a health resource for stress and well-being in a stressful working environment (González-Siles et al., 2022). SOC was investigated in relation to work stress and well-being perceived by care professionals. The review indicates that stress, depression, burnout and post-traumatic stress disorder are negatively associated with SOC; in contrast, job satisfaction, well-being and quality of life are positively associated with SOC.

SOC and Implication in Healthcare Practice

The concept of SOC can play an influential role in the meeting, communication and building of a relationship with patients and their significant others in practical healthcare. The concept of SOC provides a good foundation for delivering the right care for the right patient (Figure 2.6). Patients with low SOC are likely to have several risk factors and problems, which necessitates a greater need for interventions that should be implemented even before, for example, a treatment and with long-term planning and follow-ups.

It should be emphasised that high SOC does not exclusively mean that all situations in life are comprehensible, manageable and meaningful. Rather, it means that situations significant to the individual are perceived as such. For one individual, having a large social network may not be important, but close relationships are, on the other hand, important. For another individual the reverse may apply, but both have high SOC. A high degree of SOC is the basis for successfully handling a stressful situation. It is not an attribute of

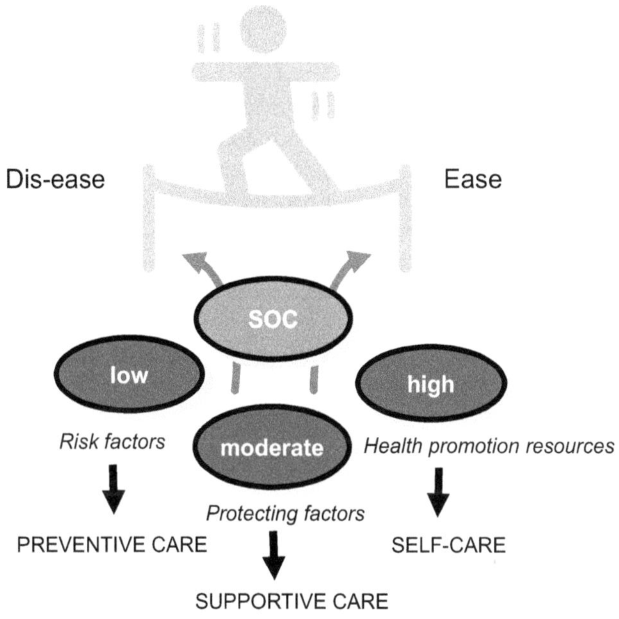

FIGURE 2.6 SOC-degree and need for supportive care actions here.

Illustration created with Canva.

happiness, as a person with a disease may be happier than a person who is healthy. Nor should a person be valued by their degree of SOC, as it is not a matter of being a good person or a less good person.

It is not the responsibility of healthcare professionals to change a patient's personality characteristics such as the degree of SOC but rather to recognise those who are vulnerable and in need of support to mobilise their own resources. The use of the scale for assessing SOC is not yet routinely implemented in clinical practice. One contributing factor is that effective application requires a deeper theoretical understanding to prevent misuse or misinterpretation – such as labelling patients as "better" or "troublesome." The knowledge of the patients' degree of SOC is indicative when planning treatment, care and rehabilitation in an individual manner. Assessment can be performed in the meeting with the patients in a conversation and integrated as a foundation for supportive actions to sustain health and well-being, as illustrated in the following cases (Box 2.1 and Box 2.2).

BOX 2.1 CASE HIGH SOC

Lisa, 51 years old, is married, has two children under the age of 15, and works as an advertising consultant when she is diagnosed with diabetes. Lisa was aware that she was at risk of developing diabetes because both her mother and grandmother have the condition. She has always tried to maintain a healthy diet and exercise regularly. When Lisa began experiencing frequent thirst, urination and unusual fatigue, she promptly sought medical attention. The doctor referred her to a nurse-led diabetes clinic, where she participated in a five-week educational programme. Lisa took time off work on the days the course was held and stated that receiving the diabetes diagnosis gave her additional motivation to further improve her diet and exercise habits.

Analysis

Lisa has several health-promoting factors that are likely to help her manage her diabetes well and avoid complications. She expresses a desire to cope with her new situation and feels motivated to manage it, based on her understanding of the challenge and her belief that she has the resources to handle it. Lisa is assessed as having a high level of SOC, which contributes to good adaptation to the diabetes diagnosis.

With the right support, a person with low SOC may begin to take greater control over their life. Over time, this support might not only prevent further weakening of their SOC but could even contribute to strengthening it. This means that the care of individuals with actual poor or threatening health conditions cannot be performed according to a single routine applicable to all. It must be recognised that patients have different ways of coping with the situation based on their degree of SOC. It is a cornerstone in the salutogenic perspective to emanate from a humanistic view where personal experience and

BOX 2.2 CASE LOW SOC

Astrid, 51 years old, is single and unemployed. Her father has diabetes. Astrid is overweight and, since becoming unemployed last year, has started drinking large amounts of alcohol at weekends. She often feels thirsty and drinks beer to quench her thirst. One day, while visiting the employment office, which she does regularly, she appears so pale and tired that the staff immediately refers her to a physician. After an examination, Astrid is diagnosed with diabetes and is offered the same educational programme as Lisa. Astrid attends the first and second sessions but then stops coming. She stays at home, has developed depression, and wonders why this has happened to her. She thinks she will never get a job now: "Who would want to hire a diabetic?"

Analysis

Astrid has few health-promoting factors available to her and does not understand why this has happened, despite knowing that she is at risk of developing diabetes. She struggles to manage the situation and finds little meaning in it. She does not view illness as a challenge worth investing effort in. Astrid has many risk factors contributing to her situation and needs support in dealing with them. However, some health-promoting factors can be identified, such as regularly visiting the employment office and following the advice to book an appointment with a physician. These may be more effective to strengthen than focusing solely on the risk factors. Astrid is assessed as having a low level of SOC, which means that she requires individual support in addition to standard patient education to adapt to the diabetes diagnosis.

perceptions are in focus. It is crucial in encounters with patients to consider each individual's ability to manage stressful situations. In each encounter, healthcare professionals need to reflect on how to make a situation comprehensible, manageable and meaningful (Box 2.3) and see how it can be improved for the patient (Box 2.4).

BOX 2.3 HOW CAN AN ENCOUNTER BE COMPREHENSIBLE, MANAGEABLE AND MEANINGFUL FOR A PATIENT?

Comprehensibility

- give knowledge that the patient understands
- information should be clear and repeated as needed
- communicate openly and honestly

Manageability

- provide resources to support the patient
- strive to create a sense of participation
- give feedback
- convey a sense of security

Meaningfulness

- encourage patients in a positive spirit
- convey motivation
- show a willingness to care

BOX 2.4 HOW CAN A SITUATION BE IMPROVED FOR A PATIENT?

- Start from the person's health resources and ability to comprehend, manage, and find meaning.
- Interventions should be tailored to each individual to avoid setting unattainable goals. For someone with a lower SOC, goals may need to be smaller and approached incrementally, for example, by, first maintaining function, and then gradually improving it.
- Strive to achieve the agreed goals. Otherwise, chaos may arise for both individuals with both a high and low SOC. Regardless of a person's degree of SOC, a situation characterised by a low SOC may be created.

Summary

The concept of SOC based on a salutogenic approach to health offer a perspective that builds on patients' strengths and coping capacities. This perspective deepens the understanding of human complexity and life orientation, providing both scientific insight and practical relevance. A person's overall ability to cope with illness and disease plays a significant role in shaping health outcomes and well-being. In encounters with patients, it is relevant to identify health-promoting resources and to determine how a situation can be made comprehensible, manageable and meaningful for each individual. In addition to identifying health-promoting resources and exploring ways to improve a situation, it is essential to tailor actions based on patients' degree of sense of coherence, ensuring that the goals pursued are realistic and attainable. Designing healthcare interventions with a salutogenic approach can improve patient support by considering their resources that promote health and well-being, rather than focusing solely on disease. In Chapter 3, learning during illness is explored as an ongoing process, focusing on how patients' learning relates to learning theories.

References

Antonovsky, A. (1979). *Health, stress, and coping*. Jossey-Bass.

Antonovsky, A. (1987). *Unraveling the mystery of health: How people manage stress and stay well*. Jossey-Bass.

Dymecka, J., Gerymski, R., Machnik-Czerwik, A., Derbis, R., & Bidzan, M. (2021). Fear of COVID-19 and life satisfaction: The role of the health-related hardiness and sense of coherence. *Frontiers in Psychiatry*, 12, Article 712. https://doi.org/10.3389/fpsyt.2021.712103

Eriksson, K. (1984). *The idea of health* [*Hälsans idé*]. Almqvist & Wiksell.

Eriksson, M., & Mittelmark, M. B. (2017). The sense of coherence and its measurement. In M. B. Mittelmark, S. Sagy, M. Eriksson, G. F. Bauer, J. M. Pelikan, B. Lindström, & G. A. Espnes (Eds.), *The handbook of salutogenesis* (pp. 97–106). Springer.

González-Siles, P., Martí-Vilar, M., González-Sala, F., Merino-Soto, C., & Toledano-Toledano, F. (2022). Sense of coherence and work stress or well-being in care professionals: A systematic review. *Healthcare*, 10(7), Article 1347. https://doi.org/10.3390/healthcare10071347

Haring, R., Feng, Y. S., Moock, J., Völzke, H., Dörr, M., Nauck, M., Wallaschofski, H., & Kohlmann, T. (2011). Self-perceived quality of life predicts mortality risk better than a multi-biomarker panel, but the combination of both does best. *BMC Medical Research Methodology*, 11, 103. https://doi.org/10.1186/1471-2288-11-103

Lazarus, R. S., & Folkman, S. (1984). *Stress, appraisal, and coping*. Springer.

Lindblad, C., Langius-Eklöf, A., Petersson, L. M., Sackey, H., Bottai, M., & Sandelin, K. (2018). Sense of coherence is a predictor of survival: A prospective study in women treated for breast cancer. *Psycho-Oncology*, 27(6), 1615–1621. https://doi.org/10.1002/pon.4702

Mittelmark, M. B., Sagy, S., Eriksson, M., Bauer, G. F., Pelikan, J. M., Lindström, B., & Espnes, G. A. (Eds.). (2017). *The handbook of salutogenesis*. Springer.

Saboga-Nunes, L., Bittlingmayer, U., & Okan, O. (2019). Salutogenesis and health literacy: The health promotion simplex! In O. Okan, U. Bauer, D. Levin-Zamir, P. Pinheiro, & K. Sørensen (Eds.), *International handbook of health literacy: Research, practice and policy across the life span*. Policy Press. https://doi.org/10.51952/9781447344520.ch042

Sajjad, A., Freak-Poli, R. L., Hofman, A., Roza, S. J., Ikram, M. A., & Tiemeier, H. (2017). Subjective measures of health and all-cause mortality: The Rotterdam Study. *Psychological Medicine*, 47(11), 1971–1980. https://doi.org/10.1017/S0033291717000381

Sundberg, K., Nilsson, M., Petersson, L. M., Kenne Sarenmalm, E., & Langius-Eklöf, A. (2022). The sense of coherence scale in a clinical nursing perspective: A scoping review. *Journal of Clinical Nursing*, 31(11–12), 1428–1439. https://doi.org/10.1111/jocn.160

World Health Organization. (1986). *Ottawa charter for health promotion*. https://www.paho.org/en/documents/ottawa-charter-health-promotion

World Health Organization. (1946). *Constitution of the World Health Organization*. https://www.who.int/about/governance/constitution

3

LEARNING DURING ILLNESS

Lena Engqvist Boman

Do you ever find it difficult to inform patients? If so, is it because patients don't remember or understand the information, because they have received too much or contradictory information, because they don't want to know, or for other reasons? If you have experienced any of these difficulties, especially patients not remembering or understanding, you share it with many other healthcare professionals as well as with patients and their relatives.

Receiving information is not the same as understanding it. The focus needs to shift from simply providing information to using principles of learning to support patients in understanding and managing their situation. This chapter concerns learning in general and what and how patients learn during illness and their experiences related to theories and concepts of learning. It also provides an opportunity to reflect on your previous experiences when you have learnt something and/or supported someone else's learning. Before you continue reading, you might want to stop and think about what learning means to you.

Learning in General

Learning encompasses content, what is to be learnt; the learning process, how the content is learnt; and the learning outcome. For example, if you are going to learn how to cook a new dish, the content is the recipe: understanding what ingredients are included, how to handle them and how to cook the food. The process is how you go about learning to cook the dish. You might start by reading the recipe and, after purchasing all the ingredients, start following the instructions step by step. You need to use certain tools in the kitchen and if you are not familiar with them, you need to learn how they work. To find a balance among the ingredients, you may need to taste the dish and adjust it. The content for learning thus includes both theoretical and practical knowledge. The learning process involves reading, thinking, perhaps asking and/or observing someone cooking the food, and using all the senses – smell, taste,

DOI: 10.4324/9781003540861-4

sight and touch – to get feedback on the outcome: does it taste good or not? The learning outcome is that you theoretically and practically understand how to cook the dish, how it tastes and what others think of it. This illustrates that the learner needs to be involved in taking in and processing information with all senses if possible, and by thinking, reacting, comparing new information with what they already know, testing and applying the new knowledge. The content, process, feedback and outcome when learning to cook a new dish are illustrated in Figure 3.1.

Learning is more complicated than Figure 3.1 suggests. The literature shows that it is a multifaceted and complex phenomenon that cannot be explained by one single theory and that there is no generally accepted definition of the phenomenon. Learning is considered to encompass not only the acquisition of skills and understanding but also the development of competence and ability to cope with various challenges in life, such as illness. A brief overview of some theories of knowledge and learning is presented in the following section, as they have had a significant impact on many educational systems and the perception of learning. The selected theories of learning in this chapter rest on a constructivist paradigm, in which the learner is viewed as an active participant processing information cognitively, emotionally and through practice, individually and in interaction with the environment and/or others, to create understanding and manageability (Illeris, 2009b; Lincoln et al., 2011).

Theoretical Perspectives on Learning

The view of knowledge and learning has developed since ancient times in various scientific fields such as physiology, biology, psychology, philosophy and sociology. The philosophy of the ancient Greeks, Plato and Aristotle, has influenced the development of education at European universities. Aristotle divided knowledge into three forms: episteme (factual knowledge, knowing what), techne (practical knowledge, knowing how) and phronesis (practical

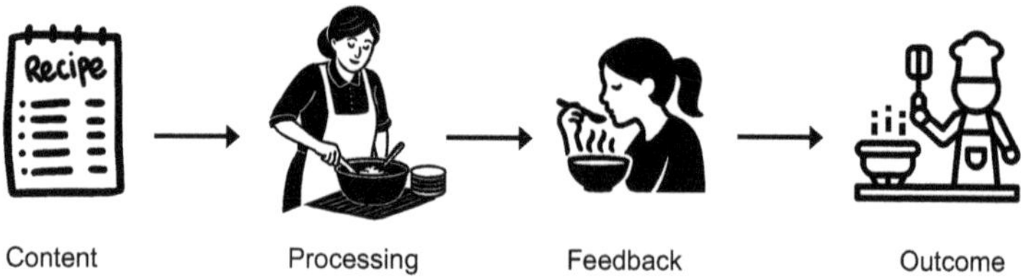

FIGURE 3.1 The elements of learning to cook a new dish – content, process, feedback and outcome.

Illustration created with Canva.

wisdom, knowing when and why). These forms of knowledge still exist in university teaching in Europe and could be transferred to patients' learning.

Modern learning theories have been developed since the early 20th century, starting with the behaviourists Pavlov and Skinner. They demonstrated how individuals learn new behaviours through conditioning such as reward, punishment and association between stimuli (Pavlov's dog). Their research has had a major impact on education, as has the work of the psychologist Piaget, who focused on children's learning related to their cognitive development while Vygotsky focused on children's learning related to social interactions. The well-known pedagogy of "learning by doing" was introduced by the philosopher John Dewey and has also greatly influenced education. Dewey emphasised that students need to learn by experiences and develop knowledge which is useful in their professional and private lives. Knowles et al. (2005) introduced a model of adult learning which is in line with Dewey's philosophy. Adult learning includes six core principles:

1. Adult learners need to know why, what and how
2. The self-concept of the learner includes the need to be autonomous and self-directing
3. Prior experience of the learner includes resources and mental models including habits, prejudices and preconceptions
4. Readiness to learn is related to life and developmental task
5. Orientation to learning is problem-centred and contextual
6. Motivation to learn is based on intrinsic value and personal payoff

Knowles believes that all groups of adult learners will be heterogeneous and that greater emphasis in adult education must be placed on individualising teaching and learning strategies. This is also true concerning adult learning during illness. This means that every patient must be treated as a unique individual with unique needs.

To create a comprehensive understanding of learning, Illeris (2009a) presented a model based on theories from psychology, biology and social science. All learning, according to Illeris, involves internal and external processes. The internal psychological processes of the learner are the focus of behaviourist and cognitive learning theories, and the external interaction between the learner and the environment is the focus of the social learning theories. The internal and external processes of learning were brought together by Illeris into a comprehensive model that describes an integrated interaction between three dimensions of learning:

1. Incentives for acquisition of the content
2. The individual's manageability
3. Interaction between the environment and the individual

The dimension of incentives includes drivers such as emotions, motivation and will to learn, aiming for mental balance of the learner (Illeris, 2009b; Mezirow, 2009). Content is what is learnt from various sources of information: a book, a lecture, a conversation, an observation, an experience, written information, instructions, practice, etc. In the acquisition of the information, the learner constructs meaning and ability to develop functionalities to manage new challenges in life. The learning includes an interaction between the learner and someone or something that contributes to learning in the situation. Drivers for learning are the individual's motivation and need for meaningfulness and trust in the learning situation. Learning during illness shares many features with learning in general but also has special characteristics to consider.

What do you think is the difference between learning in general and learning as a patient?

Learning During a Breast Cancer Trajectory – A Case Study

Research on patient learning is rare. Most studies have focused on patients' needs for and satisfaction with information and education from healthcare professionals. Taking a learning perspective is fundamental to understand not only what content patients need but also how learning occurs and can be facilitated. The learning process during a chronic illness varies both between individuals and within individuals (Kneck et al., 2014). Special circumstances for learning exist during illness, as the patient is forced to learn about their disease, treatment, self-care and coping with a situation which is potentially both threatening and unfamiliar. As an example of what this might mean, the first part of this section presents a study on women's experiences of learning during treatment for breast cancer. In the second part, the findings from the study are discussed in relation to the selected theories of learning to deepen understanding of the phenomenon.

An interview study was performed with women treated for primary breast cancer about their experiences of learning during the disease and treatment (Engqvist Boman et al., 2017). The findings are described below in relation to the content, process and outcome of learning.

Content of Learning – Multiple Sources

The study showed that the women needed to interact with large amounts of information from many sources (Figure 3.2). In addition to the information

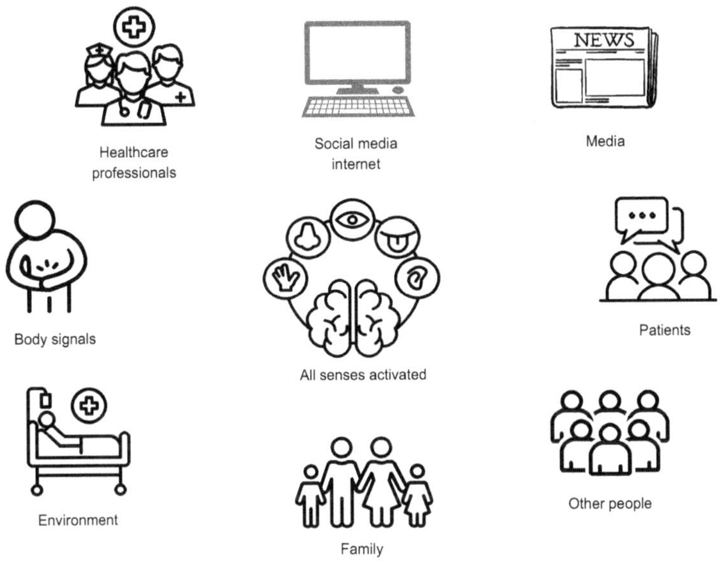

FIGURE 3.2 Sources of learning content during illness.

Illustration created with Canva.

they received from healthcare and their own search for information, they also needed to deal with information from sources they did not control, such as their body and events within and outside healthcare. These sources turned out to be very important in the process of creating understanding.

Intentional information such as the oral, written and practical information given by healthcare professionals was greatly appreciated. The various forms of information and the healthcare professionals answering questions and checking the understanding of the patients greatly supported their learning. However, extensive, irrelevant, frightening and sometimes contradictory information was a barrier to learning. The women searched for information from many sources, such as the internet and in conversations with healthcare professionals, other patients, family and friends. The sources on the internet were found to be helpful to fill information gaps. These concerned, for instance, detailed information about the disease and treatment, body appearance after breast reconstruction, cancer prevention, dietary advice and how to talk to children about cancer. Some women searched for as much information as possible and tried to sort out the most relevant. Sometimes, however, the information was frightening and hindered further searching. Sharing the breast cancer experience with others was appreciated by some women but was avoided by others who did not want to identify themselves with the disease or talk about it.

Unintended information came from the women's perceptions of bodily sensations and from being part of events within and outside the healthcare system. All senses were activated, and body and mind absorbed and interpreted stimuli from bodily sensations and events in an ongoing process. Examples of information that the senses absorbed were seeing one's own ultrasound images of the breast, hearing numbers mentioned during radiation treatment, smelling chemotherapy, feeling changes in the skin or in the taste of food, perceiving pain or nausea, and one's own or others' palpation of the breast. Other examples of unintentionally obtaining information were through participating in events, including watching TV, seeing or hearing about others' experiences with cancer, and noticing sudden changes in healthcare professionals' behaviour. The latter can be exemplified by a quote from a woman who realised, based on the behaviour of the nurses and radiologist in the X-ray room, that she had cancer. She said: "This may sound completely absurd, but I noticed that the nurses in the room and the radiologist were suddenly behaving differently and one of the nurses put a hand on me, so I thought – shit, then it really is cancer" (Engqvist Boman et al., 2017, p. 798, R7).

Learning Process – An Ongoing Struggle

The learning process was characterised by an ongoing struggle of grasping and processing the information to understand and manage the many different situations in daily life and during treatment and care (Figure 3.3). Important elements in this meaning-making process were the women's pre-understanding, motivation to learn, time for reflection and talking with family, friends and sometimes other women with breast cancer, and dialogue with the healthcare professionals when questions arose.

The pre-understanding includes knowledge, thoughts, experiences and self-understanding. The latter influenced the women's attitudes towards learning, life and how they managed their situations. Women with a high need for control adopted an approach of searching for all the information they could get. If the women were satisfied with the information provided by the healthcare professionals, the need to seek information elsewhere was reduced. An example of how pre-understanding could affect understanding was a woman who knew there could be many side effects from the anti-hormonal treatment she was receiving, but she had none of them. She said: "These stiff joints and sweating and stuff – if you don't get these reactions, is that normal, could it mean something, am I reacting too little?" (Engqvist Boman et al., 2017,

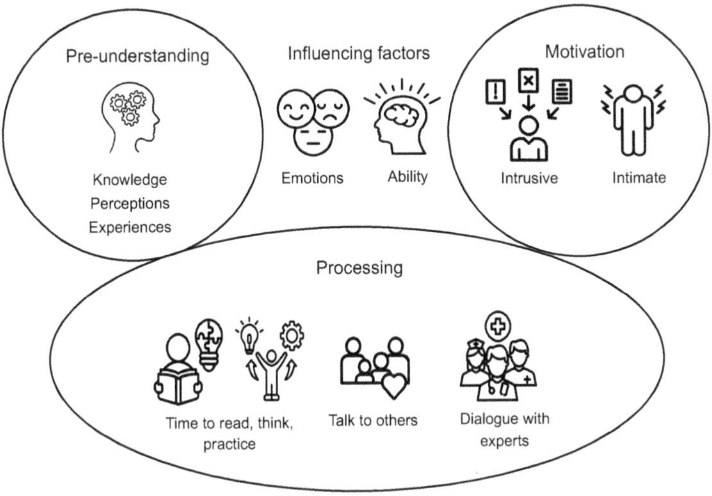

FIGURE 3.3 Learning process during illness.

Illustration created with Canva.

p. 800, R4). Because of the woman's pre-understanding about the anti-hormonal treatment, she interpreted her lack of reaction as meaning that the treatment was not effective. If this were true, why should she take the medicine? If it were not true, she needed to know that the treatment worked even without side effects.

The motivation to learn was both intimate and intrusive because the women could not choose to learn about their illness and treatment but were forced to do so to manage their health and well-being, which was threatened. Before surgery, the intrusive drivers to learn were to understand how to prepare for the operation and for participating in decision-making about treatment and research studies. Other examples of intrusive drivers were the need to understand the expected bodily effects of treatment and self-care. Body sensations before, during and after treatment were intimate drivers behind learning and searching for information. The aim was to understand and take control over one's well-being and do something on one's own, like "What can I do? How can I help here?" Some wanted to get information directly and not be wrapped in a hope that did not exist. This facilitated the process of mental preparation for the treatment. The drivers for learning changed over time depending on what was considered to be the most relevant information in the current situation.

The women needed time for reflection and dialogue with healthcare professionals and others. In the dialogue, opportunities for questions and feedback were requested, which facilitated decision-making and self-care. Having access to a contact nurse with designated responsibility for the patient at the hospital was of great importance, as the women could contact and/or visit the nurse to check physical symptoms and ask questions when they needed to. Support from nurses and doctors was particularly important when conflicting information about treatment options was provided, making it difficult to understand and decide which options were best. Sometimes it was difficult to formulate questions for the doctor during the consultation – "You know what to ask after you leave the room."

Emotions played an important role in how women perceived information, both what was communicated and how it was communicated. Verbal and nonverbal information could be delivered in a calm and positive manner that conveyed hope. When it was presented in an unclear, insensitive or dramatic way, such as: "Do you know that you have a very serious illness?" the women became frightened. Other obstacles to understanding were reduced attention at diagnosis and the perceived impaired memory due to the crisis and treatment. It took time to assimilate and process the information both cognitively – "What did they say, what does it mean?" – and emotionally – "Help, I'm going to look mutilated!"

The women's ability to process information and their emotions affected their learning and thus their ability to participate in big or small decisions about their treatment and care. Most women felt they did not have enough knowledge about the best treatment or how they would feel after surgery and therefore preferred that experts make the decisions for them. Feelings of shock and despair also made decisions difficult.

Learning Outcomes – Three Dimensions of Understanding

The learning outcomes concerned three dimensions: cognitive understanding, emotional understanding and manageability. These dimensions of understanding concerned all aspects of the illness and treatment, including care and their own situation.

All women cognitively understood that they had been diagnosed with breast cancer, but their understanding varied greatly. Some were able to describe their specific cancer in detail; others were able to name the type and/or stage of the breast cancer. Some patients understood only that their cancer was "bad" or "good," even though it was not clear to them what it meant.

Emotional understanding was related to the women's pre-understanding. Whether they had previously had a good or bad experience with cancer influenced their emotional understanding. Sometimes the emotional understanding of losing control dominated, resulting in distrust of their own bodies. If the doctor instilled hope, emotional understanding dominated even if the type of cancer was of the "worst" kind. However, conflicting cognitive and emotional dimensions of understanding complicated the overall understanding.

Manageability concerned self-care including participation in their own care.

An important part of the learning process was a changed understanding of oneself and one's own life, which included both cognitive and emotional understanding and manageability of the new situation. Physical changes due to surgery and chemotherapy, such as loss of energy, breasts or hair, and side effects of antihormones such as depression, dry mucous membranes and joint pain, were all described as affecting understanding, sometimes expressed as "I don't recognise myself." For some, the experience of breast cancer contributed to personal development and changes in their lives.

The women's interpretation of information from any of the above-mentioned sources could either be concealed or expressed to those around them (Figure 3.4). Concealed understanding emerged as an important finding, especially since misunderstandings could not be detected. This means that the women did not show their understanding in any way, that others did not notice it or that the women themselves were not aware of it. Sometimes the women intentionally concealed their understanding because they wanted to protect others, including healthcare professionals. Understanding could also be concealed unintentionally, such as when women misinterpreted symptoms or a situation and did not contact healthcare professionals for help or information. When being part of events in healthcare, the women were highly aware of what was happening. The healthcare professionals' verbal and non-verbal expressions were interpreted, and sometimes the women understood that they had cancer before anyone told them. A shocking realisation that she had cancer hindered the woman's ability to listen and was perceived "as a sudden filter" that blocked the ability to assimilate the following information. When the women did not show their understanding through emotional or verbal expressions, or when the healthcare professionals did not pay attention to it or understand the women's interpretation, communication broke down. An example of concealed understanding was an 83-year-old woman who felt sad and did not have the energy to spend time with friends as she did before antihormone treatment. She wanted to stop taking the medication but hesitated, and when asked why she did not, she said: "If I stop taking this anti hormone treatment, will I get any help and support if I relapse?" (Engqvist Boman et al., 2017,

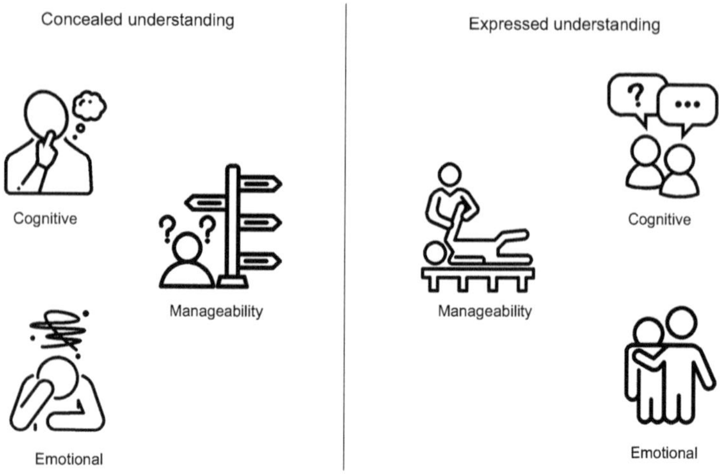

FIGURE 3.4 Learning outcomes during illness.

Illustration created with Canva.

p. 799, R14). This illustrates a misunderstanding that was never discovered by the physicians and nurses and that hindered the woman from deciding about her treatment and well-being.

When women expressed their understanding through talking, showing emotions or skills, it became possible for the healthcare professionals to detect and confirm and/or correct misunderstandings. The cognitive understanding was expressed verbally during consultations with the healthcare professionals, in emails or in patient-prepared written questions. Emotional expressions such as crying, showing anxiety or worry were other ways of showing understanding. Expressed manageability was the women's demonstration of their skills, such as palpating their breasts or massaging their arm to relieve lymphedema, and they needed feedback from the healthcare professionals. As an example, a 90-year-old woman wanted to visit the physiotherapist after returning home from hospital. She wanted to show how she did the arm exercises that the physiotherapist had instructed her to do. The physiotherapist did not consider it necessary because the woman was performing the exercises correctly before she was discharged from hospital. She also wanted to spare the woman the trouble of travelling to the hospital, also considering her age. However, the woman insisted: "I want to come and show you anyway," which she did, and was very satisfied after receiving feedback that she had done the exercises correctly.

Do you recognise any of the experiences described above in patients you encounter in your daily work?

Patients' Experiences Related to Concepts and Theories of Learning

In this section, patients' experiences of learning during breast cancer treatment and care, as presented above, are related to concepts and theories of learning. These concern pre-understanding, motivation, meaningful and transformative learning, variation for learning, and learning through the lived body. Although the concepts and theories are discussed in relation to the breast cancer case, they can be transferred to other diagnoses or health conditions. All patients, whether they have risk of disease, non-life-threatening disease (appendicitis, hip replacement, hearing problems, vertigo), chronic disease (diabetes, rheumatism, heart failure) or life-threatening disease (metastatic cancer, trauma, cardiac infarction), need to be seen and understand their situation.

Pre-Understanding

Pre-understanding is based on an individual's knowledge, experiences, assumptions and beliefs, from which new understanding is actively constructed (Illeris, 2009b). It is necessary for processing what is to be learnt. Pre-understanding shapes this process and leads to variation in understanding between individuals. Through pre-understanding, patients interpret their illnesses, symptoms and experiences, as well as information provided by healthcare professionals and other sources.

For women with breast cancer, bodily sensations and participation in events were important sources of understanding. These were interpreted in relation to pre-understanding and strongly shaped understanding. This was illustrated in how the women explained their disease and treatment, for example, the causes of their breast cancer and side effects, and in how a new lump in the breast could be interpreted as benign, like previous lumps. Self-understanding was also an important aspect of pre-understanding and influenced how the women approached learning and life, and how they dealt with their situation. Those who described a strong need for control tended to seek as much information as possible about how to improve their well-being. Those who were satisfied with the information received from healthcare felt less need to seek information elsewhere. Healthcare professionals were not always aware of what constituted the content of the women's learning, for example, what they experienced through bodily sensations or participation in events. Their pre-understanding and interpretation of information were not apparent when the women did not express them. To facilitate patients' learning, making their pre-understanding visible is therefore important, as is making visible the pre-understanding of healthcare professionals.

> *How can you make the patient's pre-understanding visible? How can you make your own pre-understanding about the patient visible?*

Motivation

Motivation of the individual for, and ability to, acquire information and interaction with the environment are basic elements in how the learning proceeds (Illeris, 2009a; Marton & Booth, 1997; Mezirow, 2009). Unlike student learning, patient learning is forced upon the individual when diagnosed with a disease, as shown in the example of getting breast cancer. The motivational factors for learning are therefore both intrusive and intimate because they affect the individual's body and life situation. For women with breast cancer, these factors included, for example, the need to know what the body would look like when the breast was removed or replaced by an implant, how to deal with side effects of treatment, how to prevent cancer recurrence, how to improve one's well-being and how to talk to family and friends, but sometimes also one's chances of survival. The motivation to learn concerned the individual's entire life situation related to physical, psychological and sociological needs.

Motivation has been distinguished between extrinsic and intrinsic motivation (Ryan & Deci, 2000). Extrinsic motivation responds to external demands such as rewards or compulsion to learn while intrinsic motivation represents the drivers such as curiosity and strong will to learn within the learner. The latter has proved to result in high-quality learning, while learning from external drivers varies in quality. However, extrinsic rewards can transform learners' engagement and turn it into an internally rewarding learning process (Bardach & Murayama, 2025). The external demands on patients to learn are high, as shown in the breast cancer study. The women were forced to absorb and process substantial information in a short period to understand what the diagnosis and treatment meant and how it would affect their lives. This is not in line with supporting learning, which means starting from the patient's needs, questions and concerns that could be seen as the internal motivational factors. Supporting students as learners, to enhance their feelings of competence and autonomy, is assumed to increase their motivation and self-determination (Ryan & Deci, 2000). The same support to patients also needs attention. The internal demands can facilitate learning as "I need to know how to manage the side effects" and the healthcare professionals can help. Feelings of stress and anxiety are other internal motivational factors for understanding and gaining control over the situation but can also inhibit the ability to learn. The external demands may engage patients' internal driver to learn as it may increase their control of the situation and well-being. Sometimes the motivation to understand is ambiguous, as described by a woman who both wanted and did not want to know about survival rates. This illustrates that a serious illness like breast cancer raises questions of life and death, but that does not necessarily mean one is ready to learn about and deal with such questions. The motivation for learning shifted in relation to the individual, the current situation and what the patient considered relevant to understand at that time. Because patients' needs and motivation to learn change over time, healthcare professionals must continuously and carefully assess these needs.

Have you ever been forced to learn something? What was it like? Think of something you enjoyed learning! What motivated you? How did it affect your learning?

Meaningful Learning

Meaningfulness is closely related to motivation to learn and to understanding the content and situation for learning. Meaningful learning is always connected to a social context (Marton & Booth, 1997). An individual's understanding of a phenomenon differs between reproducing knowledge and seeking meaning of what is learnt. Meaningful learning, in short, can be described as the learner receiving, understanding and using information and being able to transfer the knowledge to other situations. This contrasts with rote learning, which means that the learner remembers facts but does not understand them and cannot use or transfer them to another situation (Mayer, 2002). Patients are not expected to be able to repeat information without understanding it. However, there is a great risk of this when patients receive substantial information in a short time. It is not uncommon for them not to remember or understand everything they have been informed about. The variation in understanding of their disease was found in the breast cancer study, where some had in-depth knowledge of their cancer type while others only knew that they had a bad or good cancer. Those with in-depth knowledge had often sought information themselves, in contrast to those who did not know much about their breast cancer. Furthermore, if the social context and the medical language are unfamiliar to the patient and there is a power imbalance between patients and healthcare professionals, it can hinder meaningful learning if no one asks patients about their need for knowledge. In addition, patients need time and support to process information, practical instructions and their experiences related to their illness and treatment by, for example, being asked to explain its meaning and demonstrate their skills.

The content of learning needs to be relevant for, and coherent with, the unique current needs of the patients, which vary during the course of a disease. If the information is not relevant, the information is forgotten. For example, when a woman with breast cancer received information about a breast prosthesis that was not relevant to her because only part of her breast was to be removed, she did not pay attention to the information. Later the entire breast was removed anyway, and by then she had forgotten the information about the prosthesis.

The need for information varies between individuals. Some women in the breast cancer study were satisfied with the information they received from healthcare providers. Others searched for and wanted all the information they could get to choose the most relevant. The relevance of the content is one of the most important drivers for meaningful learning, as pointed out by Knowles et al. (2005) and Marton and Booth (1997), among others. Therefore, the relevance of the learning content needs to be attended to in healthcare.

How do you know if the learning content is relevant and meaningful to patients? How do you assess their cognitive and emotional understanding, skills and manageability?

Transformative Learning

For some women, the experience of having breast cancer meant a changed outlook on life. For example, they prioritised other things in life such as family over work and doing things that made them feel happy. The women's experiences can be compared to the theory of transformative learning presented by Mezirow (2009). It means that individuals construct meaning from their experiences and through their frames of reference. Transformative learning includes the individual's critical reflection on their own and others' assumptions, leading to changed beliefs and actions based on the new understanding. This can be exemplified by women with breast cancer who used critical reflection on doctors' assumptions, assessed and compared information from different sources, including research, about treatment with antihormones and questioned its relevance. To make decisions about treatment, the women needed a dialogue with their doctors about the effects and side effects of the anti-hormonal treatment and the consequences if they discontinued the treatment. If this need was not met, the women became uncertain and worried about their decisions. This highlights the role of the healthcare professionals as facilitators of patients' learning. A space for reflection and dialogue seems necessary to support the understanding of the patients (Engqvist Boman et al., 2017; Johansson et al., 2016; Kneck et al., 2014).

How do you and your team/colleagues meet patients who have a different opinion about their treatment than the one recommended?

Learning Through Variation

In the theory of variation, learning is described as the discernment of something different, which is captured by the individual's awareness (Marton & Trigwell, 2000). This is exemplified by women who perceived something new in the body, such as a lump in the breast, skin sensitivity after radiation or pain from chemotherapy. When the information from the body did not agree with the information received from healthcare, it caused anxiety and confusion. The women did not understand what was happening or how to deal with their bodily sensations. Sometimes the women did not contact the nurse at the hospital as they thought the nurse could not help. Instead, they tried out solutions on their own, for instance, what to eat when everything had a disgusting taste. According to the theory of variation and that bodily sensations vary between women, and for a long time after treatment completion, one could argue for giving information about all variations of side effects to all women. However, since the driving force for learning is the perceived discernment of something new and learning is supported by the relevance of the content (Marton & Booth, 1997), this creates a dilemma. The dilemma is that the women need to be prepared to manage their situation for a long time after treatment is completed but need the information only when it is relevant and they perceive something new in their body or well-being. This means that patients need to know whom they can contact within healthcare who can meet their needs for information and support, sometimes even for an extended period.

The theory of variation can also contribute to shedding some light on women's perceptions of the surroundings. Changes in the behaviour of the staff during a clinical consultation are variations which are interpreted by the women. Examples of such variations are when the staff suddenly starts to talk with a soft or childish voice, tilting the head, patting the woman's head or mumbling when examining the breast. These variations were noted by the women, who interpreted them as signs of having breast cancer. Sometimes this was correct and sometimes not. The interpretation caused anxiety, which hindered the women from assimilating further information. If the women concealed their interpretations, no one could pay attention to them. Feedback could not be given until the women expressed their understanding verbally or emotionally. This exemplifies the significance of the patient's interaction with the healthcare professionals to get support during the learning process. The healthcare professionals may not be aware of their own behaviours or how they are interpreted by the patients. In addition, the awareness of the women is not always directed to the same content of learning as the one the healthcare professionals are aiming for, and meaningful learning is not supported (Marton & Booth, 1997). Awareness of differences in the current situation needs to be addressed by healthcare professionals to facilitate patients' understanding.

Do you have an example of when you "discovered" something new that stimulated you to try to understand? What was the trigger for your learning? How can you detect if the patient has experienced something in their body or environment that they are worried about?

Learning Through the Lived Body

Another important source of learning was the women's perceptions of their own bodily sensations, which were interpreted in relation to their pre-understanding. The findings can be understood in relation to the phenomenology of perception presented by Merleau-Ponty (2002). He states that learning about the world is to perceive and process a variety of stimuli through the body and to internalise the new understanding as a part of oneself. He also argues that the body is not an object that can be understood in its parts. All parts are intertwined, and there is no other way to learn about the world than to perceive it through the body, of which the brain is a part.

Leder (1990) agrees with the view that it is through the body we live and learn, called the Lived Body. When the body is functioning, it is not noticeable and, in that sense, it disappears from our consciousness and is what he calls the Absent Body. When the body is not functioning, it reveals itself to our mind, which he calls a dysfunctional and dys-appeared body. Pain, disease and social breakdown are examples of when the body dys-appears. It can be exemplified by women who perceived a filter blocking their ability to hear what was said, after they had received their breast cancer diagnosis. The inability to hear could be described as a "dys-appeared body," that is a dysfunctional body which comes to the fore of the individual's awareness and makes it impossible for the women to hear the following information. If this is ignored by those who provide the information, it will not be assimilated by the patient. Another example of a 'dys-appeared body" was a woman who perceived that she belonged to the 5%, who got all the bad things. Several times, before the surgery as well as the adjuvant treatment, she was informed that she probably would not get the unusual treatment, as only 5% of all women got it. After the examinations of her breast tissue, it turned out that she needed the unusual treatment. She understood she could not trust her body anymore – it had disappeared from her control – and wanted someone else to tell her if she was healthy or not. It can be assumed that the intention of healthcare professionals in informing patients about the most common treatment is to convey hope and trust. However, as demonstrated in the previous example, it had the opposite effect and contributed to feelings of distrust of the body and perhaps also to the information delivered by the staff.

Both Merleau-Ponty and Leder argue that the body is not an object that can be understood in its parts, in contrast to the Cartesian view of body and soul as divided parts. Leder, who is a physician, believes that the latter has affected the encounters between patients and healthcare professionals when patients feel treated as a "thing." Instead, he believes that one should uncover concealed phenomena and pay more attention to the patient's experience and subjective voice to promote their healing. It was very clear in the breast cancer study that the women collected and interpreted information with all senses activated in an ongoing process. Sometimes they concealed their understanding from the healthcare professionals, and hence misunderstandings could not be detected. Healthcare professionals must be aware of the ongoing learning process and pay attention to what patients experience both in their bodies and surroundings, but also how patients interpret and understand these experiences.

> *How can you help patients express their concealed understanding?*

Summary

Theories and concepts of learning related to research on patient learning contribute to our understanding of how learning occurs during illness. A summary of learning during illness is presented in Box 3.1. All learning takes time, and

BOX 3.1 SUMMARY OF LEARNING DURING ILLNESS

Patient Learning Is

- an ongoing process over a long period
- characterised by strong emotions

Patients

- are overwhelmed by information, with all senses involved
- receive information from healthcare, bodily signals and the surroundings
- learn through variation in bodily signals and the behaviour of others
- are compelled to learn because it concerns their body, health and life

Patients Need

- understandable and relevant information suited to the current situation
- support in expressing their needs and pre-understanding
- time to think, talk to others and practise skills in order to process information
- opportunities to ask questions and receive answers from experts
- feedback on their understanding, skills and ability to manage
- understanding in order to participate in their care

Patients'

- needs for information and understanding differ between individuals
- needs for information and understanding change over time
- pre-understanding affects their understanding of new information
- experience may involve a changed view of themselves and of life

for patients it is an ongoing process during diagnosis, treatment and rehabilitation and sometimes throughout the rest of their lives. The body plays a crucial role because all senses are involved in collecting and interpreting information in a constantly ongoing process. The content is more than the information delivered from healthcare, and information from all sources must be considered, especially body signals and information from the surroundings. The patient's ability, emotions, motivation and perception of what is relevant to learn in the current situation influence the process. Patients need time to process all information and their experiences and emotions in interaction with others such as family, friends, other patients and healthcare professionals. The outcome of learning differs between patients depending on their needs, preunderstanding and interpretation of information from the different sources. The content, process and outcome of patients' learning need to be addressed to facilitate their understanding and management of their situation. Chapter 4 will present the concept of health literacy and its relevance for patients' ability to access, understand, appraise and apply health information to promote health and well-being.

References

Bardach, L., & Murayama, K. (2025). The role of rewards in motivation: Beyond dichotomies. *Learning and Instruction*, 96, 1–11. https://doi.org/10.1016/j.learninstruc.2024.102056

Engqvist Boman, L., Sandelin, K., Wengström, Y., & Silén, C. (2017). Patients' learning and understanding during their breast cancer trajectory. *Patient Education and Counseling*, 100(5), 795–804. https://doi.org/10.1016/j.pec.2016.12.024

Illeris, K. (2009a). A comprehensive understanding of human learning. In K. Illeris (Ed.), *Contemporary theories of learning: Learning theorists . . . in their own words* (1st ed., pp. 7–20). Routledge. https://doi.org/10.4324/9780203870426

Illeris, K. (Ed.). (2009b). *Contemporary theories of learning: Learning theorists . . . in their own words* (1st ed.). Routledge. https://doi.org/10.4324/9780203870426

Johansson, K., Österberg, S. A., Leksell, J., & Berglund, M. (2016). Patients' experiences of support for learning to live with diabetes to promote health and well-being: A lifeworld phenomenological study. *International Journal of Qualitative Studies on Health and Well-Being*, 11(1). https://doi.org/10.3402/qhw.v11.31330

Kneck, Å., Fagerberg, I., Eriksson, L. E., & Lundmand, B. (2014). Living with diabetes-Development of learning patterns over a 3-year period. *International Journal of Qualitative Studies on Health and Well-Being*, 9(1), 11–12. https://doi.org/10.3402/qhw.v9.24375

Knowles, M. S., Holton III, E. F., & Swanson, R. A. (2005). *The adult learner* (6th ed.). Routledge. https://doi.org/10.4324/9780080481913

Leder, D. (1990). *The absent body*. University of Chicago Press.

Lincoln, Y. S., Lynham, S. S., & Guba, E. G. (2011). Paradigmatic controversies, contradictions, and emerging confluences, revisited. In N. K. Denzin & Y. S. Lincoln (Eds.), *The SAGE handbook of qualitative research* (pp. 97–128). SAGE.

Marton, F., & Booth, S. (1997). *Learning and awareness*. Erlbaum.

Marton, F., & Trigwell, K. (2000). Variatio est mater studiorum. *Higher Education Research & Development*, 19(3), 381–395. https://doi.org/10.1080/07294360020021455

Mayer, R. E. (2002). Rote versus meaningful learning. *Theory Into Practice*, 41(4), 226–232. https://doi.org/10.1207/S15430421TIP4104_4

Merleau-Ponty, M. (2002). *Phenomenology of perception* (Original work published 1945). Routledge.

Mezirow, J. (2009). An overview on transformative learning. In K. Illeris (Ed.), *Contemporary theories of learning: Learning theorists . . . in their own words* (1st ed., pp. 90–105). Routledge.

Ryan, R. M., & Deci, E. L. (2000). Intrinsic and extrinsic motivations: Classic definitions and new directions. *Contemporary Educational Psychology*, 25(1), 54–67. https://doi.org/10.1006/ceps.1999.1020

4

HEALTH LITERACY

Josefin Wångdahl

Do you find that patients do not always follow your advice? That they are well-informed – but about the wrong things? That they rely on inaccurate health information? Or that they return repeatedly without having improved their health?

During an illness these circumstances may be related to limited health literacy, which, in essence, refers to the ability to access, understand, appraise and apply health information. Health literacy is not the same as general literacy, which relates to a person's ability to read and comprehend written information. Nor is it the same as health knowledge, which, somewhat simplified, concerns factual understanding of health-related topics. This chapter introduces the concept of health literacy and focuses on three key questions: What is health literacy? Why is it important for individuals and society? And how can health literacy be addressed in healthcare?

Expectations of Patients and Their Exposure to Health Information

In today's society, individuals – including patients – are increasingly expected to have basic health knowledge and the ability to seek relevant health information. They are also expected to take the initiative to make informed decisions, live healthy lives and take responsibility for their own health, including performing appropriate self-care. However, it can be difficult to navigate the vast amount of health information available today. Some information is actively sought by individuals in response to specific health problems, for example, by searching the internet, contacting health advisory services, or consulting family members or friends. At the same time, individuals passively receive a substantial amount of health information. This can occur in everyday conversations with neighbours, for example, or through various media such as

DOI: 10.4324/9781003540861-5

television, radio, newspapers and online platforms. It can also be obtained from food packaging and various types of advertising.

In other words, people in today's society have access to a wide range of health information from many different sources – not only from the healthcare sector (Figure 4.1). This can be seen as positive, as it can promote knowledge and facilitate informed decisions, but it also poses challenges, as not all health information comes from sources that are primarily focused on promoting health. Some actors, such as commercial companies, may prioritise the sale of health-related products and services, which can lead to the spread of misinformation or disinformation – for example, misleading claims about the effects of certain dietary supplements or treatments. Furthermore, the information that patients encounter is not always relevant to their personal situation, and it is not always reliable or evidence based.

Therefore, it is important that we all have a sufficient level of health literacy, which, somewhat simplified, can be described as an individual's ability to access, understand, appraise and apply health information in a way that promotes health (Sørensen et al., 2012). A patient having those abilities is more likely to access information and identify which information is trustworthy and useful, helping them to make informed choices about their care. In contrast, patients with limited health literacy may struggle to access information and evaluate the credibility or relevance of health information they encounter. Consequently, this increases the risk of acting on misleading or incorrect information, which may ultimately harm their health.

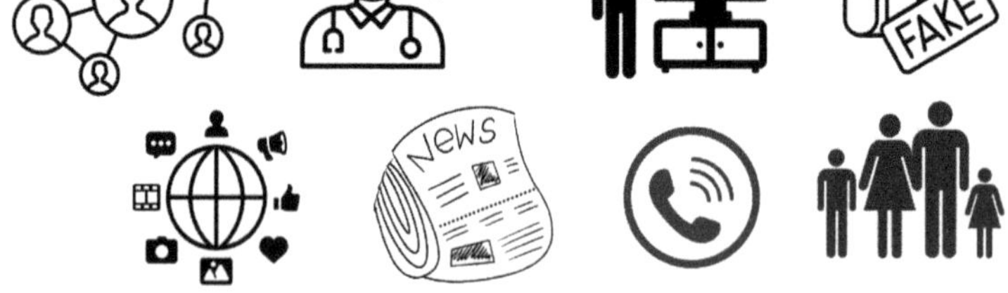

FIGURE 4.1 Various sources of health information.

Illustration created with Canva.

Health Literacy at the Individual Level

Several definitions and dimensions of health literacy at the individual level exist. Recognising that different forms of health literacy exist – and that the concept may carry slightly different meanings – is important for understanding how health literacy can be applied in diverse contexts.

In this text, the term "health literacy" refers specifically to general health literacy at the individual level. This is because general health literacy represents the broadest and most inclusive form of health literacy.

The World Health Organization (WHO, 2021) defines health literacy as "personal knowledge and competencies that accumulate through daily activities, social interactions and across generations. Personal knowledge and competencies that are mediated by the organisational structures and availability of resources that enable people to access, understand, appraise and use information and services in ways that promote and maintain good health and wellbeing for themselves and those around them."

Another widely used definition, by Sørensen et al. (2012), states that health literacy at the individual level is "linked to literacy and entails people's knowledge, motivation and competence to access, understand, appraise, and apply health information in order to make judgements and take decisions in everyday life concerning healthcare, disease prevention and health promotion, in order to maintain or improve quality of life during the life course."

Most definitions of health literacy share a common understanding: it describes a person's ability to use health information and consists of more or less the same core competencies (Box 4.1). What mainly distinguishes them is the variation in terminology and the number of competencies included. Other differences include the types of health information referred to, and whether the definition emphasises that health literacy is context dependent (Sørensen et al., 2012).

BOX 4.1 HEALTH LITERACY SIMPLIFIED

In simplified terms, individual health literacy can be described as a person's ability to access, understand, appraise and apply health information in order to make decisions that promote health.

The Core Competencies of Individual Health Literacy

The four core enabling competencies that collectively shape and influence an individual's overall level of health literacy (Sørensen et al., 2012) are outlined

below. Understanding these competencies can provide a clearer picture of what it means to have high or low health literacy. Furthermore, it can help to understand how health literacy can be assessed and what efforts are important to focus on to facilitate people with limited health literacy levels and promote health literacy.
Accessing information (Figure 4.2) is about knowing where to turn to obtain various forms of health information that you or someone else needs. For example, it is about knowing and being able to contact your country's healthcare advice service, your healthcare centre or another organisation or person that has knowledge about health. This can also be a caregiver or someone in your own social network. Several different skills may be needed to access health information today, for example, reading, using the internet, and computers.

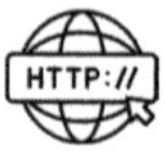

FIGURE 4.2 Accessing information.

Illustration created with Canva.

Understanding information (Figure 4.3) means being able to understand written information, for example, patient education materials, notices, medicine leaflets and lists of ingredients on food packaging. Further, it means being able to understand oral information, for example, what health and care professionals, relatives, newsreaders and others say.

FIGURE 4.3 Understanding information.

Illustration created with Canva.

Appraising information (Figure 4.4) involves evaluating the health information you receive to determine whether it is credible, reliable and relevant to you. While this may seem self-evident when accessing information through mass media or the internet, it is equally important when receiving health information from relatives or others in society. This is because of the vast amount of health information available from various sources – and the fact that many myths and misconceptions persist about health, healthcare and caregiving.

FIGURE 4.4 Appraising information.

Illustration created with Canva..

Applying information (Figure 4.5) means being able to use health information in a timely, relevant and appropriate manner. This process also requires several of the previously mentioned health literacy skills. For example, to take medicine as prescribed, you need to correctly use the information and instructions provided, understand them, and, if necessary, ask questions to clarify any uncertainties.

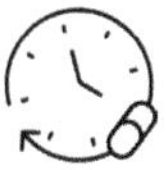

FIGURE 4.5 Applying information.

Illustration created with Canva.

Dimensions of Individual Health Literacy

Another common theoretical approach, defined by Don Nutbeam, focuses on three dimensions of individual health literacy: functional, communicative and critical health literacy (Nutbeam & Lloyd, 2021).

Functional health literacy (Figure 4.6) relates to a large extent to a person's ability to read and use written health information so that they can, for example, read and understand information about an appointment or a packet of medication. This also includes being able to understand numbers and do simple calculations, for example, to work out how much medicine to take.

FIGURE 4.6 Functional health literacy.

Illustration created with Canva.

Communicative health literacy (Figure 4.7), sometimes also referred to as interactive health literacy, relates to a person's cognitive and social abilities to select and communicate about health topics with others based on the current situation. For example, being able to tell health professionals about how you feel and how your body feels so that they can understand what your problem is and provide the right treatment.

FIGURE 4.7 Communicative health literacy.

Illustration created with Canva.

Critical health literacy (Figure 4.8) refers to a person's ability to analyse and use information to better control different life events and situations. For example, a person's ability to assess and determine which health advice from the internet and social media, different organisations, and from family and friends is accurate and relevant. Furthermore, critical health literacy relates to a person's knowledge of the individual and societal factors that affect their own health and the health of others and the ability to influence these factors.

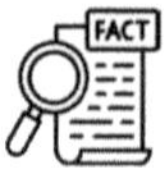

FIGURE 4.8 Critical health literacy.

Illustration created with Canva.

Historically, the focus has been on functional health literacy, which is sometimes referred to as "just" health literacy. However, over the past decade, a paradigm shift has occurred towards the broader and more complex concept – general health literacy – which includes all three dimensions: functional, communicative and critical health literacy.

BOX 4.2 HEALTH LITERACY PATIENT CASES

Case 1: Sara is a 38-year-old woman with chronic migraines who communicates effectively with her healthcare provider. She asks detailed questions, shares relevant experiences and carefully considers treatment options in relation to her lifestyle. However, she has difficulty understanding written medical materials and often relies on verbal explanations from her doctor.

This means that Sara has *low functional health literacy* because she struggles to understand written information. However, she demonstrates *high communicative health literacy* by discussing her health effectively with her provider, and *high critical health literacy* by analysing information and making informed decisions about her care. Although Sara has l*ow functional health literacy*, her *overall health literacy is relatively high* because her strong communication and critical thinking skills help her manage her health effectively.

Case 2: John is a 60-year-old man with diabetes who is highly skilled at finding and understanding medical information online. He regularly researches his condition, medications and treatment options, and follows written guidelines to manage his diabetes effectively. However, he struggles to ask questions or express concerns during medical visits and often leaves without fully understanding his treatment. He also has difficulty critically evaluating online information and tends to accept it without questioning its reliability or relevance.

This means that John has *high-functional health literacy*, as he is adept at finding and understanding health-related information online and following written instructions. However, he has *low communicative health literacy* because he does not actively engage with his healthcare provider, and *low critical health literacy* because he does not critically evaluate the information he encounters. Although John has *high-functional* health *literacy*, his *overall health literacy is relatively limited* because difficulties with communication and critical evaluation may hinder informed healthcare decisions.

A person can have different levels of functional, communicative and critical health literacy. For example, someone with low functional health literacy but high communicative and critical health literacy may still demonstrate relatively good overall health literacy. Conversely, a person with high-functional health literacy but low communicative and critical health literacy might have limited general health literacy. However, there is ongoing discussion in the literature about whether these three dimensions should be seen as progressively advanced levels that build on one another. For instance, some argue that functional health literacy may be a prerequisite for developing communicative and critical health literacy. Box 4.2 uses two patient cases to explain this.

Thus, health literacy at the individual level is much more than the ability to read and understand information. It is linked to literacy but not the same. Moreover, it is not the same as knowledge and comprehension alone. Health literacy is action-oriented and enables people to constantly engage with new and changing information during the life course.

Digital Health Literacy

In addition to general individual health literacy, there are several more specific subtypes. These focus either on the source of health information – such as digital health literacy – or on a particular health topic, for example, mental health literacy. The significant increase in digital information and health services in society has made digital platforms a central part of how individuals seek, receive and manage their health-related knowledge and care.

General health literacy and digital health literacy are strongly related, and both include the ability to access, understand, evaluate and use health information to make informed decisions (Levin-Zamir et al., 2025). However, digital health literacy focuses more specifically on digital sources and resources for health information that is accessed through digital platforms, while also adding the interactive skills and abilities that are unique to the digital setting. This is reflected in the definition by the WHO Action Network on Measuring Population and Organizational Health Literacy (M-POHL, 2021), describing digital health literacy as

> the ability to search for, access, understand, appraise, validate, and apply online health information, and to formulate/express questions, opinion, thoughts, or feelings when using digital resources.

Thus, digital health literacy is not only about the ability to navigate digital environments. It also involves evaluating digital health information sources, such as health apps, social media and online platforms. In addition, it includes the ability to make informed individual choices. These competencies are becoming increasingly important as digitalisation expands, and health information and resources become more widely available in society (Levin-Zamir et al., 2025).

Theoretical Frameworks and Models for Individual Health Literacy

Over the years, several theoretical frameworks and conceptual models for individual (general) health literacy have been developed. While they vary in specific details and areas of emphasis, they all share common foundational principles regarding the significance of health literacy. These frameworks aim to define what health literacy is and place it within a broader healthcare and societal context. Additionally, they illustrate the factors that influence health literacy, the ways it affects individuals and systems, and the dynamic relationships between these elements. Examples of commonly used frameworks and models are the integrated model of health literacy by the European Health Literacy Consortium (Sørensen et al., 2012), Paasche-Orlow & Wolf's Casual Pathway model of health literacy (Paasche-Orlow & Wolf, 2007), Baker's conceptual model of health literacy (Baker, 2006), Nutbeam's outcome model for health promotion (Nutbeam, 2000) and Parker's Health Literacy Framework (Parker, 2009). They all in various ways try to explain what affects and what is affected by health literacy.

Below, the integrated model of health literacy by the European Health Literacy Consortium is presented in more detail (Figure 4.9). This model adopts a holistic approach and is grounded in a comprehensive review of existing definitions and frameworks of health literacy that were conducted in 2012. It is one of the most thorough models available, making it a valuable tool for understanding health literacy as a relational concept focusing on the individual and the interaction with information, services and stakeholders involved in healthcare, disease prevention and health promotion.

The model provides a comprehensive overview of health literacy – what it is, what influences it and how it affects health outcomes. At its centre is the core of health literacy: the knowledge, motivation and competencies needed to access, understand, appraise and apply health information to make informed decisions about healthcare, disease prevention and health promotion in everyday life. It shows, on the one hand, how individuals – whether healthy, at risk or ill – can manage their health, seek support and navigate healthcare services to support their quality of life. On the other hand, it illustrates the interaction with organisations and stakeholders, for example, health professionals, who enable how well people can access, understand, appraise and apply information and services to manage health matters related to healthcare, disease

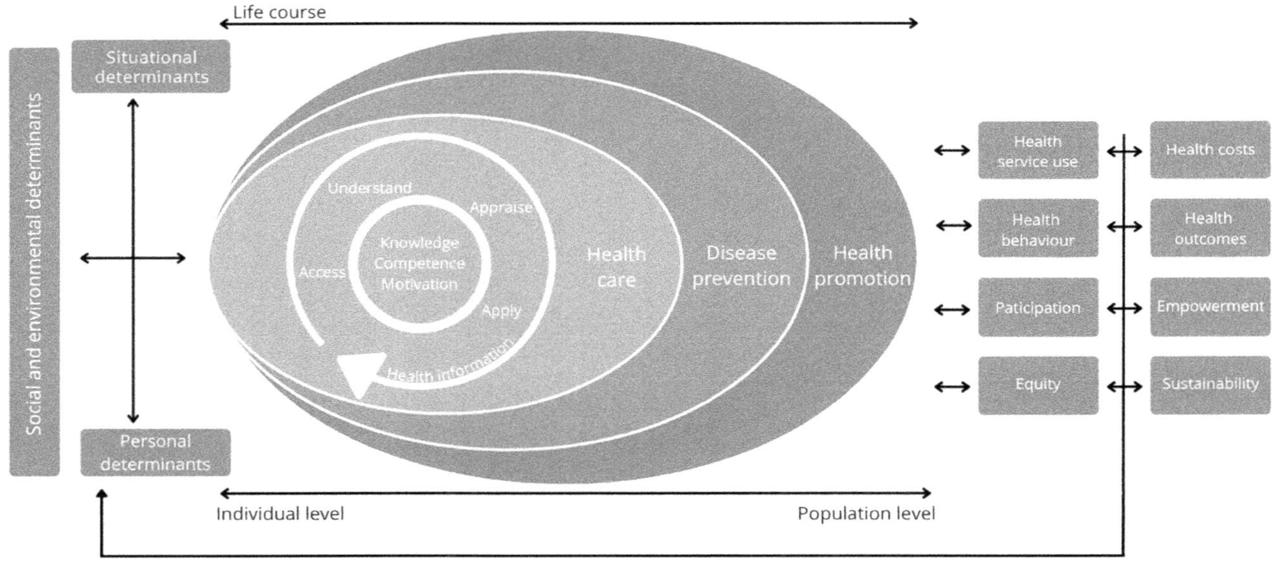

FIGURE 4.9 The integrated model of health literacy.

Illustration created with Canva and is based on a figure by Sørensen et al. (2012)

prevention and health promotion. Health literacy evolves over the course of life and can be influenced and changed depending on situation and context. In this regard, the model indicates how health literacy is influenced by personal factors like age, gender, education, socio-economic status, language, beliefs and traits such as shyness or self-esteem. Situational factors including living and working conditions, social support and surroundings as well as societal factors like environment, culture and social systems.

In addition, the model illustrates that health literacy both influences and is influenced by various outcomes, including health service utilisation, healthcare costs, health behaviours and overall health status. It also shapes how individuals engage with their health and empowers them to take control of it. Importantly, health literacy contributes to reducing inequalities and promoting sustainability – both at the individual level and through systemic impacts on healthcare and beyond. Finally, the model shows that these outcomes are interconnected and affected by the same factors that determine an individual's health literacy.

QUESTIONS FOR REFLECTION

- What is the difference between literacy and health literacy?
- How can a person have relatively high general health literacy even if functional health literacy is low?
- How can a person have relatively low general health literacy even if functional health literacy is high?
- What are the differences and similarities between individual and organisational health literacy?

Why Health Literacy Is Important

Health Literacy and Health Outcomes

Research consistently shows that health literacy is linked to a range of health outcomes. For example, individuals with limited health literacy are more likely to misunderstand health information, make decisions based on incomplete or incorrect knowledge, and struggle to follow medical instructions (Berkman et al., 2011; van der Gaag et al., 2022). One illustration of this is a patient who takes all prescribed medication in the morning instead of splitting the dose between morning and evening, or who stops treatment early because they feel better, without realising the importance of completing the full course. These misunderstandings can lead to ineffective treatment, worsened symptoms or complications.

Individuals with limited health literacy are also less likely to understand the importance of health promotion and tend to participate less in disease prevention (Berkman et al., 2011; van der Gaag et al., 2022). The reason why people do not participate in screening is partly due to a lack of knowledge or misunderstanding about how it works. For example, parents who believe that the human papillomavirus (HPV) vaccine for young girls is administered in the genital area rather than in the arm are less likely to have their daughters vaccinated. Misinformation and rumours like this can significantly influence health decisions. During the Covid-19 pandemic, for instance, people with limited health literacy were less likely to follow public health advice regarding hand hygiene, social distancing and the use of face masks (Hermans et al., 2021).

Further, health literacy influences decision-making related to health and how individuals use healthcare services (Berkman et al., 2011; M-POHL, 2021). For example, individuals with limited health literacy visit general practitioners more frequently, experience longer hospital stays and have slower recovery after surgery. It is also more common that they avoid seeking care when it's needed. This could be due to difficulty recognising symptoms or uncertainty about when and where to seek help. As a result, care can be delayed until the condition becomes more serious and requires more advanced treatment.

A somewhat counterproductive finding is that individuals with limited health literacy often ask fewer questions (Menendez et al., 2017). This may happen because of the shame and embarrassment related to having limited literacy, which can make patients afraid to seem uninformed. Another reason can be that they do not know what questions to ask or fear being a nuisance. Further, people with limited health literacy more often have unhealthier lifestyles, that is, eat less healthily and are more physically inactive, and have poorer health status (physically and mentally) (Berkman et al., 2011; M-POHL, 2021).

In summary, limited health literacy is associated with a range of negative health outcomes, while adequate health literacy can help prevent unnecessary illness, reduce the severity of disease and shorten the duration of ill health. Sufficient health literacy, on the other hand, increases individuals' ability to understand and use health information to make informed decisions and take an active role in one's care (Berkman et al., 2011; Ghorbanian Zolbin et al., 2022; van der Gaag et al., 2022).

Health Literacy in the Chain of Care

Health literacy plays a critical role throughout every stage of the chain of care. Figure 4.10 illustrates how health literacy influences a patient invited to a health screening aimed at preventing disease and promoting health, such as mammography or some form of vaccination.

Before the healthcare encounter, the first challenge related to health literacy is understanding the invitation and any accompanying information about the screening – some of which may have been received passively through friends or media. Patients may also need to actively seek additional information and assess its reliability to make informed decisions. Limited health literacy can lead to confusion, misunderstanding and reliance on inaccurate sources, potentially resulting in declined participation and missed opportunities for early detection. In contrast, sufficient health literacy supports understanding of the purpose of screenings and encourages participation, which can lead to early identification of health issues and preventive action.

During the healthcare encounter, patients need to comprehend the information provided, express their concerns clearly and ask questions when needed. It is also helpful if they can reflect on whether the diagnosis or treatment aligns with their symptoms and situation. Limited health literacy may cause misunderstandings, hinder communication and contribute to missed or incorrect diagnoses. Adequate health literacy, on the other hand, improves dialogue between patients and providers and supports more accurate identification of health problems and active patient involvement.

After the healthcare encounter, it is beneficial if patients are able to critically reflect on the support and treatment they may have received, follow the agreed-upon medical advice and treatment instructions, and seek out and evaluate additional information relevant to their condition. Limited health literacy can lead to poor understanding, decisions based on incorrect or insufficient information, and low adherence to treatment, which may reduce the effectiveness of care. In contrast, adequate health literacy supports well-informed decision-making, appropriate use of health information and contributes to improved health outcomes.

Health Literacy at the Population Level

According to European surveys on individual health literacy conducted in 2011 and again between 2019 and 2021, nearly one in two individuals in Europe exhibit limited health literacy (Sørensen et al., 2015; M-POHL, 2021). Both surveys involved large sample sizes, with thousands of participants across seven European countries. In most countries, data were collected through surveys in the language of the majority population, which means that migrants

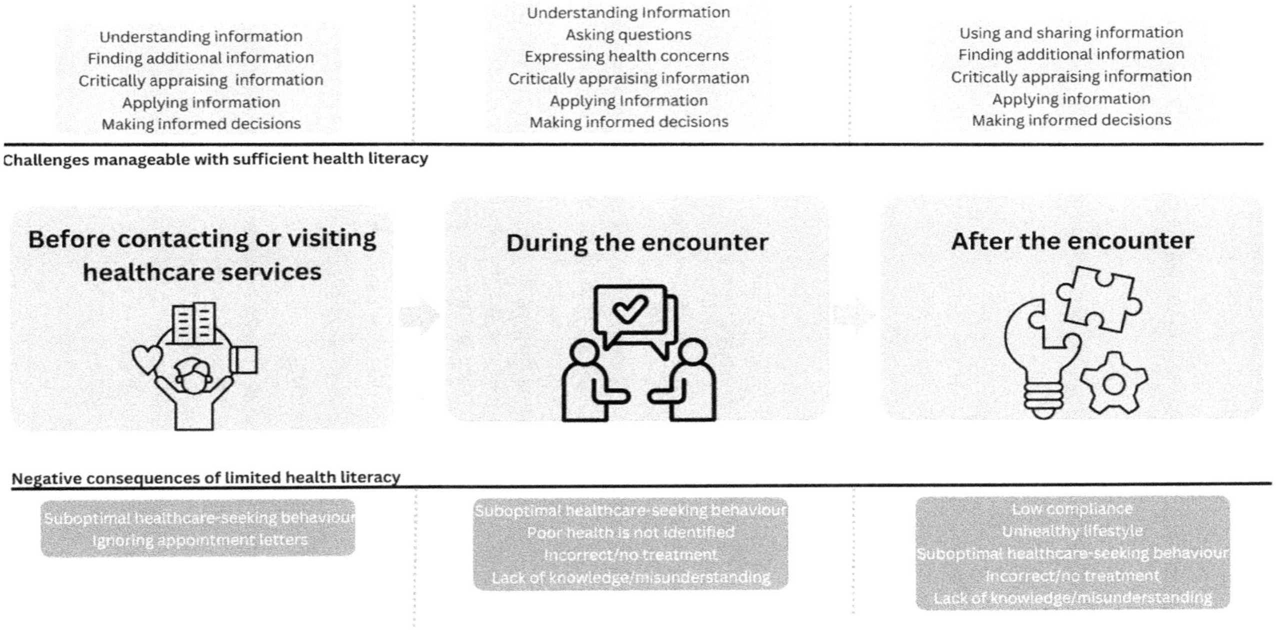

FIGURE 4.10 Health literacy in the chain of care.

Illustration created with Canva.

with limited skills in that language probably did not participate and are therefore underrepresented in the study. While limited health literacy exists across all segments of the population, those and several other studies have also shown it is more prevalent among certain subgroups:

- individuals with low levels of education
- people with low socio-economic and/or social status
- migrants
- older adults

This is important to highlight, as it shows that limited health literacy exists across the entire population. Moreover, language proficiency is just one of many factors influencing an individual's health literacy level. Although this has been discussed earlier in the chapter, it bears repeating, as the misconception that health literacy is mainly a language issue can lead to underestimating patients' actual abilities.

Assessment of Individual Health Literacy

There are many different instruments available to measure health literacy at the individual level. These instruments are primarily developed for research and evaluation purposes and are not intended for routine use in clinical practice. One way to categorise these instruments is to divide them into performance-based instruments and self-assessment instruments. When using any instrument, it is important to select an instrument that aligns with the purpose and is appropriate for the target group. The instrument should be adequately translated and culturally adapted. Also keep in mind that some individuals may have difficulty with written questions. In such cases, oral assessment can be a useful alternative – though it may lead to overestimation of health literacy, as stigma may cause individuals to report stronger skills than they actually have.

Performance-Based Instruments

These instruments are based on the principle that individuals, whose health literacy is being assessed, perform tasks that require, for example, reading comprehension, numeracy or knowledge of medical terminology. The more correct answers, the higher the individual's health literacy is considered to be. Most performance-based instruments assess specific aspects of health literacy. Examples of such instruments are the Newest Vital Sign (NVS), test of functional health literacy in adults (TOFHLA) and Rapid Estimate of Adult Literacy in Medicine (REALM) (Tavousi et al., 2022).

Self-Assessment Instruments

These instruments rely on individuals' self-assessment of their own health literacy. Self-assessment instruments are applied to assess general health literacy, specific dimensions or particular types of health literacy. A common feature of these instruments is that individuals rate their own abilities – such as accessing, understanding, appraising and applying various types of health information in different situations – using a scale with predefined response options. Based on the individual's responses, a health literacy score is calculated, with higher scores indicating a higher level of general health literacy. Examples of such instruments are the European Health Literacy Survey Questionnaire (HLS-EU-Q), the Health Literacy Questionnaire (HLQ) and the Functional–Communicative–Critical Health Literacy Scale (FCCHL) (Tavousi et al., 2022).

Assessment in Clinical Practice

It is generally not recommended to use health literacy assessment instruments designed for research in everyday clinical practice. Instead, it is recommended to stay alert for possible signs of limited health literacy, such as when a patient:

- misses appointments
- seems confused by written communication
- does not follow instructions
- avoids reading provided information
- asks few questions
- nods despite not understanding

However, these signs are not definitive, as health literacy can vary by context and situation. Because it is difficult to accurately assess a patient's health literacy, it is best to apply universal precautions – communicating in a way that makes health information easy for everyone to understand and use. Clear, simple communication benefits all patients and improves care quality.

How to Work with Health Literacy in the Healthcare Sector

To reduce the potential negative consequences of limited health literacy, it is important to work at both the individual and organisational levels (Sørensen et al., 2021). Working at the individual level involves strengthening people's abilities to access, understand, evaluate and use health information in order to make informed decisions that help people to promote or maintain health and well-being. While this is most effectively achieved through schools and other educational settings, healthcare providers also play a role. For instance, healthcare providers can support patients by asking reflective questions about their sources of health information, guiding them in navigating trustworthy digital platforms, and teaching them how to interpret and use information – such as instructions on medication packaging and guidance related to self-care. However, efforts at the organisational level are even more critical. These efforts involve adapting healthcare environments, communication strategies and processes to reduce unnecessary complexity. By addressing challenges at the organisational level, healthcare services can become more inclusive, accessible and responsive to patients' needs. The goal is to make it as easy as possible for all patients – regardless of their health literacy level – to access, understand, appraise and apply health information effectively. In other words, strengthening organisations' health literacy. What this is and how it can be promoted is described in Chapter 6.

Summary

Health literacy at the individual level can be described as a person's ability to access, understand, appraise and apply health information to make decisions that promote health. In other words, it is much more than understanding written health information or possessing factual knowledge about health. A considerable proportion of the population in many countries has limited health literacy. This is critical, as health literacy is essential throughout the patient journey, and limited health literacy is linked to several negative outcomes, such as ineffective or inadequate use of health information and healthcare services, and poorer health. In evaluation and research contexts, several instruments are available to measure health literacy. In everyday clinical practice, however, the recommended approach is to remain attentive to signs of limited health literacy and apply universal precautions – making it as easy as possible for everyone, regardless of their literacy level, to access, understand, evaluate and use health information. To reduce the negative consequences of limited health literacy, it is important to work at both individual and organisational levels. This involves strengthening individuals' health literacy skills while also identifying and removing barriers that hinder people's ability to access and use health information effectively. Chapter 5 will present how a pedagogical encounter can be performed based on the concepts of sense of coherence, learning during illness and health literacy.

References

Baker, D. W. (2006). The meaning and the measure of health literacy. *Journal of General Internal Medicine*, 21(8), 878–883. https://doi.org/10.1111/j.1525-1497.2006.00540.x

Berkman, N. D., Sheridan, S. L., Donahue, K. E., Halpern, D. J., & Crotty, K. (2011). Low health literacy and health outcomes: An updated systematic review. *Annals of Internal Medicine*, 155(2), 97–107. https://doi.org/10.7326/0003-4819-155-2-201107190-00005

Ghorbanian Zolbin, M., Huvila, I., & Nikou, S. (2022). Health literacy, health literacy interventions and decision-making: A systematic literature review. *Journal of Documentation*, 78(7), 405–428. https://doi.org/10.1108/JD-01-2022-0004

Hermans, L., Van den Broucke, S., Gisle, L., Demarest, S., & Charafeddine, R. (2021). Mental health, compliance with measures and health prospects during the COVID-19 epidemic: The role of health literacy. *BMC Public Health*, 21(1), 1365. https://doi.org/10.1186/s12889-021-11437-w

Levin-Zamir, D., Van den Broucke, S., Bíró, É., Bøggild, H., Bruton, L., De Gani, S. M., Søberg Finbråten, H., Gibney, S., Griebler, R., Griese, L., Guttersrud, Ø., Klocháňová, Z., Kucera, Z., Le, C., Link, T., Mancini, J., Miksova, D., Schaeffer, D., Ribeiro da Silva, C., Sørensen, K., . . . Pelikan, J. (2025). Measuring digital health literacy and its associations with determinants and health outcomes in 13 countries. *Frontiers in Public Health*, 13, 1472706. https://doi.org/10.3389/fpubh.2025.1472706

Menendez, M. E., van Hoorn, B. T., Mackert, M., Donovan, E. E., Chen, N. C., & Ring, D. (2017). Patients with limited health literacy ask fewer questions during office visits with hand surgeons. *Clinical Orthopaedics and Related Research*, 475(5), 1291–1297. https://doi.org/10.1007/s11999-016-5140-5

M-POHL. (2021). *International report on the methodology, results, and recommendations of the European health literacy population survey 2019–2021 (HLS19) of M-POHL*. Vienna: Austrian National Public Health Institute.

Nutbeam, D. (2000). Health literacy as a public health goal: A challenge for contemporary health education and communication strategies into the 21st century. *Health Promotion International*, 15(3), 259–267. https://doi.org/10.1093/heapro/15.3.259

Nutbeam, D., & Lloyd, J. E. (2021). Understanding and responding to health literacy as a social determinant of health. *Annual Review of Public Health*, 42, 159–173. https://doi.org/10.1146/annurev-publhealth-090419-102529

Paasche-Orlow, M. K., & Wolf, M. S. (2007). The causal pathways linking health literacy to health outcomes. *American Journal of Health Behavior*, 31(Suppl. 1), S19–S26. https://doi.org/10.5555/ajhb.2007.31.supp.s19

Parker, R. (2009). Measuring health literacy: What? So what? Now what? In *Institute of medicine roundtable on health literacy, measures of health literacy: Workshop summary (Chapter 6)*. National Academies Press. https://www.ncbi.nlm.nih.gov/books/NBK45386/

Sørensen, K., Levin-Zamir, D., Duong, T. V., Okan, O., Brasil, V. V., & Nutbeam, D. (2021). Building health literacy system capacity: A framework for health literate systems. *Health Promotion International*, 36(Suppl. 1), i13–i23. https://doi.org/10.1093/heapro/daab153

Sørensen, K., Pelikan, J. M., Röthlin, F., Ganahl, K., Slonska, Z., Doyle, G., Fullam, J., Kondilis, B., Agrafiotis, D., Uiters, E., Falcon, M., Mensing, M., Tchamov, K., van den Broucke, S., Brand, H., & HLS-EU Consortium. (2015). Health literacy in Europe: Comparative results of the European health literacy survey (HLS-EU). *European Journal of Public Health*, 25(6), 1053–1058. https://doi.org/10.1093/eurpub/ckv043

Sørensen, K., Van den Broucke, S., Fullam, J., Doyle, G., Pelikan, J., Slonska, Z., Brand, H., & (HLS-EU) Consortium Health Literacy Project European. (2012). Health literacy and public health: A systematic review and integration of definitions and models. *BMC Public Health*, 12, Article 80. https://doi.org/10.1186/1471-2458-12-80

Tavousi, M., Mohammadi, S., Sadighi, J., Zarei, F., Kermani, R. M., Rostami, R., & Montazeri, A. (2022). Measuring health literacy: A systematic review and bibliometric analysis of instruments from 1993 to 2021. *PLoS One*, 17(7), e0271524. https://doi.org/10.1371/journal.pone.0271524

van der Gaag, M., Heijmans, M., Spoiala, C., & Rademakers, J. (2022). The importance of health literacy for self-management: A scoping review of reviews. *Chronic Illness*, 18(2), 234–254. https://doi.org/10.1177/17423953211035472

World Health Organization (WHO). (2021). *Health promotion glossary of terms 2021*. https://iris.who.int/bitstream/handle/10665/350161/9789240038349-eng

5

THE PEDAGOGICAL ENCOUNTER

Lena Engqvist Boman, Ann Langius-Eklöf, Kay Sundberg and Josefin Wångdahl

What works well and what do you find challenging when it comes to supporting patient learning? What skills do you have and what do you need to develop to improve your strategies to think and act patient learning?

In your daily practice, you provide patients with information and education about their condition, available treatment options and strategies for self-care. This demanding task requires healthcare professionals to possess pedagogical competence. The *Think and Act Patient Learning* framework (Figure 5.1) addresses the role of three theoretical perspectives in planning and conducting pedagogical encounters: sense of coherence (SOC), learning during illness and health literacy. The interconnections among these perspectives illustrate that patient learning is an ongoing process of understanding, developing competencies and practical skills, and finding meaning in managing situations related to illness. Unlike learning and health literacy, an individual's degree of SOC is a relatively stable prerequisite for overall coping ability throughout an illness trajectory and is therefore less sensitive to change (see Chapter 2). The framework does not aim to alter patients' SOC levels but to guide the planning of care and pedagogical encounters with the understanding that patients differ in their SOC. Although patients learn in different ways, their learning processes can be facilitated. The same applies to health literacy: patients' ability to understand, apply and critically appraise health information can be strengthened. This underscores the importance of identifying patients who need additional support to mobilise their own resources.

This chapter provides practical guidance on how you and your team can create pedagogical encounters aimed at promoting optimal patient health and well-being. It also offers opportunities to apply the knowledge from previous chapters through the *Think and Act Patient Learning* framework. The chapter covers the pedagogical role of healthcare professionals, the patient learning process, how to create a pedagogical encounter and approaches and

DOI: 10.4324/9781003540861-6

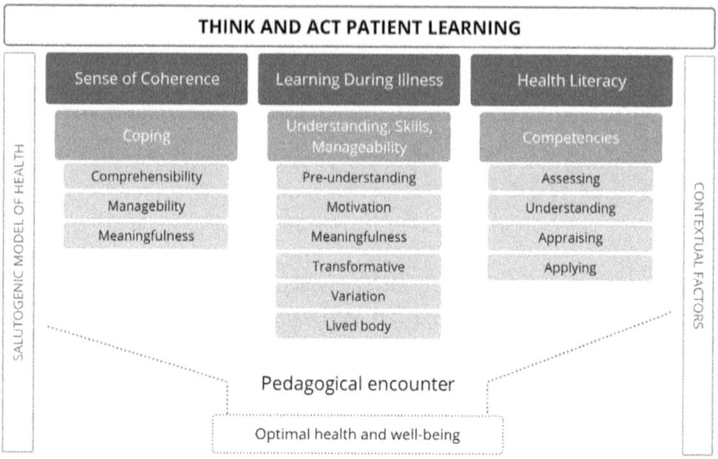

FIGURE 5.1 The *Think and Act Patient Learning* framework.

practices for supporting patient learning. It concludes with patient cases that illustrate different situations and provide opportunities to practise pedagogical encounters.

The Pedagogical Role of Healthcare Professionals

Healthcare professionals and patients share responsibility for the patient's health, and both are experts in different ways. Patients know what it is like to live with their illness. Healthcare professionals have knowledge of illness and treatment and play a crucial role in supporting patients to develop the skills needed for effective self-care. Orem's theory of self-care was originally developed to guide nursing practice, but it can be considered universal (Orem, 2001). Central to the theory is the understanding that patients are capable of, and willing to, take responsibility for their own health. The theory is structured around three key perspectives: self-care, self-care deficits and self-care systems. Self-care refers to the activities patients perform to maintain and improve their health and well-being. When a self-care deficit occurs, patients become dependent on others to help balance their self-care needs with their ability to meet those needs. Self-care systems describe different levels of support, ranging from complete care for patients in coma to educational and supportive interventions for patients who are largely self-reliant. Within the *Think and Act Patient Learning* framework, the pedagogical encounter is understood as an educational and supportive intervention. It aims to strengthen patients' self-care abilities by identifying self-care deficits and addressing them from a salutogenic perspective to promote optimal health and well-being. Although much of this book focuses on planned encounters, healthcare professionals' knowledge and competence in supporting patient learning are just as crucial in brief or unplanned encounters. Brief encounters in healthcare are often time-pressured interactions in which several important issues must be addressed within a limited timeframe. Applying theoretical knowledge to think and act in support of learning is important but may not always be feasible in every pedagogical encounter. In such situations, it becomes especially important to listen carefully to what the patient considers most important to express.

Patient education has a long history, dating back to Florence Nightingale, who taught patients how to improve their well-being to enhance health outcomes and strengthen their ability to cope with illness. Relatively few studies provide evidence on best practice in supporting patient learning, and most focus on specific conditions or clinical settings. The choice of educational method – group, individual, digital or blended – must be adapted to the situation and available resources. Structured group programmes may be suitable when the goal is to provide condition-specific knowledge, for example, in cardiac, asthma or diabetes, or when patients can benefit from sharing experiences with others living with similar illnesses. Individual pedagogical encounters, by contrast, make it possible to tailor the meeting to the patient's specific learning needs, support discussion of sensitive topics and ensure that the patient is seen and heard as a person. Focusing on patient learning is particularly important in today's healthcare system, where patients are expected to possess the knowledge and skills needed to participate in self-care. They must deal with a range of challenges, including shorter hospital stays, the digitalisation of processes such as appointment scheduling and access to information about treatments or blood tests, and shortages of healthcare professionals.

Pedagogical competence is a prerequisite for facilitating patient learning. The healthcare professional's view of, and approach to, teaching and learning plays a crucial role. Different teaching approaches can influence learning in different ways. Ramsden (2003) describes three approaches to teaching:

- Teaching as telling means that the teacher focuses on presenting and conveying content to students. The teacher does not reflect on the pedagogical aspects of teaching and "blames the students" if they do not remember or understand the content.
- Teaching as organising means that the teacher focuses on teaching techniques that activate students, such as group discussions and experiential learning processes. The teacher aims to improve teaching skills but does not necessarily adapt teaching to the students' understanding of the subject.

- Teaching as making learning possible means that the teacher focuses on students' understanding of the subject. The teacher systematically improves teaching by listening to students and other teachers and adapting learning activities accordingly. The teacher recognises that knowledge of the content is constructed by the student and that this understanding needs to be followed up.

Teaching as telling is likely to be the most common approach among healthcare professionals when informing patients about diagnosis and treatment. Teaching as organising is often used when patients are expected to learn self-care routines. Both approaches have a place in the pedagogical encounter, because patients need clear presentation of content as well as opportunities to participate in learning activities. However, to address challenges in patient learning, such as not remembering or understanding information, healthcare professionals must also adapt their practice in line with teaching as making learning possible.

Patient Learning Process

Transferring the approach of teaching as making learning possible to a healthcare context requires adopting a patient-learning perspective. In the *Think and Act Patient Learning* framework, the theoretical foundations – SOC, learning during illness and health literacy – share common elements that together form the basis for thinking in terms of patient learning. These include the patient's pre-understanding; their sense of meaningfulness and motivation to learn; perceptions through the lived body; ability to process information and experiences; understanding and manageability of their situation; skills and competencies in self-care and health-promoting resources.

The learning process begins with an individual's pre-understanding, which encompasses existing knowledge, experiences, feelings, and perceptions. Healthcare professionals therefore need to explore the patient's pre-understanding of the disease, treatment, care, and situation in relation to the health condition. New information and instructions can then be adapted to that pre-understanding, allowing a new understanding to emerge. This new understanding may contribute to a sense of meaningfulness and motivation to learn. At the same time, the motivation to learn is often imposed by the illness, and patients may feel reluctant or unable to absorb all the information they receive. Learning occurs through the lived body because all information, including bodily signals, is absorbed through the senses and interpreted by the individual, thereby creating understanding. All learning takes time, and when the interval between diagnosis and treatment is short, patients may struggle to process information, understand its content and implications, and develop manageability, practical skills and self-care competence. Processing is essential to all learning and is perhaps the most challenging aspect of patient learning. Receiving information is only the starting point; the content must be processed in various ways for the individual to develop genuine understanding (Illeris, 2009). Patients' health-promoting resources, together with opportunities to articulate their understanding, participate in discussions, practise self-care and receive feedback from experts, all contribute to learning and can increase motivation to participate actively in care. Patients need time and support to read and think through the information, discuss it with family and friends, engage in meaningful dialogue with experts, practise self-care and receive feedback on multiple occasions. Because learning is a continuous process throughout the illness trajectory, healthcare professionals across all forms of practice need to consider how best to support patients in different situations and at different times.

What strategies or ideas do you have for facilitating patients' learning process within your specific context?

Creating a Pedagogical Encounter

A pedagogical encounter in healthcare is a planned or unplanned learning situation that aims to support the patient's learning process. At its core, it involves building a relationship in a trusting environment and taking an individual approach that considers each patient's needs and ability to understand and manage their situation. The patient's development of knowledge and skills in each encounter is shaped by their pre-understanding and by how they assess, understand, value and apply information.

The structured learning situation within a planned pedagogical encounter can be applied regardless of the purpose of the meeting or the nature of the interaction with the patient. Key aspects to consider are the situation, agents, purpose, goals, intensions, interaction, content and learning activities (Silén, 2013). Integrating a salutogenic perspective into the pedagogical encounter involves recognising each patient's unique needs, competence and skills, and exploring how their situation can be made comprehensible, manageable and meaningful. Suggestions for creating pedagogical encounters in accordance with the *Think and Act Patient Learning* framework before, during and after the encounter are presented below and an overview is provided in Table 5.1.

TABLE 5.1 Overview of planning and performing a pedagogical encounter

	Before the encounter	*During the encounter*
Situation	Where will the pedagogical encounter take place? What do you already know about the patient and what are your thoughts about the patient's needs and situation?	Create a positive and safe learning environment.
Agents	Who will be participating? How will they be involved?	Introduce yourself and other agents present at the encounter.
Purpose	What will the encounter be about? Why is it important?	Declare the purpose and the scheduled time of the encounter.
Goal	What is the patient expected to understand or be able to do at the end of the encounter?	Identify learning needs collaboratively with the patient, as they may have additional or different needs than anticipated.
Intentions	What are your intentions and approach for the encounter?	Ask how the patient understands their situation and what expectations they have from the encounter. Identify individual resources that can act as facilitators in the patient's care and recovery.
Interaction	How will you start and end the dialogue, and how will you involve the patient and their relatives? How will you follow up on the patient's learning and understanding during and after the encounter?	Ask the patient what they already know, what they think about it and what questions they have. Create a dialogue, ask open-ended questions, and continuously check the patient's (and relative's) understanding after information and instructions have been given.
Content	What content, type and amount of information do you need to prepare?	Adjust the content, type, level and amount of information including practical instructions to the patient and situation.
Activities	What learning activities are you planning? How can the patient prepare for future self-care tasks?	Provide relevant and combined material, such as oral and written information and instructions of self-care. If possible, allow the patient to practice self-care, read information and reflect on it. Provide feedback on their understanding and self-care skills. At the end, inform about future plans.
After the encounter	Evaluate the encounter – ask the patient to reflect and give feedback on the performance of the pedagogical encounter. Encourage patients to read and think about the information and reflect on their self-care skills, as well as to talk to family and friends and formulate new questions. Invite the patient to contact you after the encounter if there are any more questions.	

Before the Pedagogical Encounter

You may need to prepare in several ways and reflect on your own pre-understanding of the patient and your intentions for the encounter. You need to decide where the meeting will take place, preferably in a quiet and secluded space, and how much time it will require. In addition to reading the patient's medical record, you may need to learn more about the patient's condition. The purpose of the meeting – why it is important for the patient to learn this content – and the goal – what the patient is expected to understand or be able to do by the end of the meeting – need to be clarified. You should also prepare appropriate information materials. Think through how you will start and end the meeting, how you will interact with and involve all agents, what learning activities the patient will undertake, and how you will follow up the patient's learning. Can the patient prepare in any way, for example, by writing down questions, reading recommended information, or watching an instructional video?

During the Pedagogical Encounter

In all learning situations, it is important to create a positive and safe learning environment. Establishing a trusting relationship matters and can be done by welcoming the patient and their relatives and introducing yourself, your profession, and your role. Other agents, such as students and healthcare professionals, should also introduce themselves and clarify their roles. Patients greatly appreciate healthcare professionals who are friendly and who demonstrate familiarity with their name, diagnosis, treatment and overall situation. Depending on the patient's condition, diagnosis, treatment phase, abilities and sense of coherence, they may feel more or less tense or anxious, which can affect their ability to listen, remember and understand information.

Explaining the purpose of the encounter and its scheduled duration, including time for questions, contributes to clarity and helps patients adapt and prioritise their own questions. To elicit the patient's pre-understanding, it can be helpful to ask about their expectations of the encounter and their perceptions of the situation, including their emotions. What is most relevant and important for the patient to discuss and understand right now? Learning needs should be identified collaboratively with the patient. While healthcare professionals understand what the patient must know or be able to do, for example, before treatment, the patient may have additional or different learning needs that should be acknowledged. It is equally important to recognise the individual's resources that can facilitate care and recovery. Offering different types of information and combining oral, written, visual and practical instruction can support memory and understanding. Because the content is often extensive, it helps if the healthcare professional presents information gradually, highlights the most important points and clarifies what the patient needs to do immediately. It can also be valuable to find out which sources patients rely on and how critically they evaluate them. Ask the patient to explain what they have understood and how they interpret the information. When patients verbalise their understanding, it becomes possible to confirm what they have grasped and identify gaps or misunderstandings. This can be done both during the conversation and at the end of the encounter.

If the patient is going to learn practical skills – such as administering an injection, caring for a wound or changing an ostomy bag – they need clear instructions and an opportunity to ask questions about the procedure. They also need to practise and demonstrate their ability to perform self-care, reflect on it and receive feedback through dialogue. Many individuals have limited knowledge of the human body and its functions. It is therefore important for healthcare professionals to assess not only patients' understanding of their bodies but also their experience and interpretation of symptoms and bodily signals. To invite additional concerns, it can be helpful to encourage patients to share anything that has not yet been discussed, including information they may have heard, seen or read elsewhere that is causing worry.

At the end of the meeting, a clear plan for further treatment and next steps can improve the patient's ability to manage their situation. Providing written information allows the patient to review and remember what has been discussed. Additional materials can also encourage continued learning and help the patient find answers to questions that arise later. These may include written notes, recordings made on the patient's own mobile phone, ready-made educational materials, links to relevant and evidence-based websites, and contact details for patient associations. If the next visit will take place at another unit or organisation, it is important to ensure that the patient has clear information about how to contact and get to the unit and what to expect during the visit.

After the Pedagogical Encounter

When the pedagogical encounter concludes, and before the patient leaves, it can be helpful to invite them to share feedback on how they experienced the meeting – what they found valuable, what felt meaningful and whether any part of the conversation was uncomfortable, unclear or lacking. It is also important to encourage them to explain how you or the healthcare team could better support them, including what facilitates their understanding and what could be improved to make the information clearer. Although this type of evaluation may not be feasible in every patient encounter, asking such questions from time to time can provide valuable insights and help improve your pedagogical skills. You can also improve your approach by using internal feedback: reflecting on your own experiences and discussing with colleagues what facilitated or hindered the patient's learning.

It is important that patients know whom to contact after the pedagogical encounter and how to reach them. One much-appreciated source of support is access to a nurse with particular responsibility for the patient, often called a contact nurse, who is available to answer questions and address concerns even after the patient has returned home.

Approaches for Supporting Patient Learning

In a pedagogical encounter, communication is about creating meaningful dialogue in which patients and healthcare professionals develop a shared understanding together. The goal is to establish a relationship that supports the exchange of perspectives and promotes clarity, participation and mutual respect. Focusing on the patient's perspective helps patients feel seen and heard, increases engagement, encourages questions and supports active participation in decisions about their care. Communication can be verbal or non-verbal. Words, tone of voice, facial expressions and body language all contribute to how messages are understood. For healthcare professionals, this means listening carefully to the patient while also observing non-verbal cues. For patients, it is a challenge as they not only have to interpret what is said but also how it is said. Creating accessible communication also involves practising cultural sensitivity and adopting a norm-critical approach.

Cultural sensitivity refers to recognising that people from different cultural backgrounds may have different beliefs, values and ways of behaving, and to responding to these differences respectfully and appropriately, for example, by avoiding value judgements. One way to practise cultural sensitivity is to adapt both the content and the delivery of information so that they align with the patient's cultural background. By tailoring communication in this way, healthcare professionals can promote better understanding, trust and engagement among patients from diverse cultural contexts (Jenstad et al., 2024). In practice, even small adjustments can make a meaningful difference, for example, using familiar language and culturally relevant examples, such as referring to foods commonly eaten in the patient's culture when discussing dietary recommendations.

Norm-criticism involves questioning societal norms and being aware of how they influence individuals and groups (Nye et al., 2023). In patient communication, a norm-critical approach should be applied when developing or reviewing information and educational materials so as to avoid unintentionally excluding certain groups or reinforcing discriminatory structures. Questions that may guide such reflection include:

- Which groups in the population are represented in the text and images, and which are missing?
- Which groups might feel that the information speaks to them, and which might feel excluded?
- How are people with different characteristics portrayed, for example, differences in age, gender, sexual orientation, hair, skin and eye colour, physical or cognitive variation, and socio-economic background?

In essence, communication in a pedagogical encounter should feel meaningful, supportive and comfortable for everyone involved. Each encounter should be seen not only as an exchange of information but also as an opportunity for mutual learning and reflection. By using diverse communication practices, healthcare professionals can create an inclusive and supportive learning environment (Lyu et al., 2024).

Create a Safe and Positive Learning Environment

All learning situations are unique and encompasses physical, psychological, social and cultural dimensions, each of which can have positive or negative effects on the individual's learning. The physical learning environment refers to the actual space in which learning takes place, including the room, equipment and materials used. The psychological environment concerns how the patient feels during the encounter: whether they feel calm, safe, respected and ready to take in information. The cultural environment includes the patient's background, such as language, values, beliefs and traditions, all of which can influence how they understand and respond to information and to the healthcare system. A positive learning environment is characterised by the learner's perceptions of engagement, motivation, meaningful experiences, a positive emotional climate, peer support, strong teacher-learner relationships and recognition as an individual (Rusticus et al., 2023). Patients may be highly stressed or fearful in an unfamiliar environment, or because they have had previous negative experiences of healthcare, and this can hinder learning and participation in care (Eriksen et al., 2023). The healthcare environment is not always a matter of choice and may at times be messy or even chaotic. This underscores the importance of building a trusting relationship between the patient and the healthcare professional. Patients need to feel respected, safe and recognised as unique individuals with names and identities, not merely as numbers or one patient among many. This is a basic prerequisite for participation in healthcare (Boman et al., 2018). Other important strategies include meeting the patient in a quiet and secluded space and being attentive and undisturbed by ringing mobile phones or other distractions.

> *What barriers can you identify to creating a safe and positive learning environment in your workplace? What can you do to overcome these barriers?*

Pay Attention to Attention

Do you know how long we can maintain our attention when taking in information?

Students tend to lose attention within 15–20 minutes when listening to a lecture (Biggs & Tang, 2011). When reading a textbook, attention span can vary between 10 and 120 minutes depending on the individual, the situation and the task. Patients' attention is a prerequisite for learning. The healthcare professional's strategy should therefore be to avoid a monologue and instead create a dialogue, which is necessary if patients are to maintain attention. During the pedagogical encounter, healthcare professionals need to adapt their strategies if attention drops, for example, because of strong emotions or because the information is too extensive or too difficult to understand. It is well-known that when a patient is informed of a serious diagnosis, the information can provoke anxiety and inhibit attention. As a result, patients may not hear what is said after the diagnosis, and this is sometimes described as "my hearing was turned off." Healthcare professionals must recognise that the information they provide needs to be absorbed and processed by patients who react and adapt differently depending on its amount and content. It is therefore important to give the patient space to process the information and to offer a follow-up meeting to discuss it.

> *In what situations do the patients you encounter have difficulty maintaining attention? How do you notice when a patient's attention is decreasing during an encounter?*

Support Memory

In a study in which students learned the same material in different ways, they remembered 10%–95% of the content two weeks later (Biggs & Tang, 2011). The more senses they used and the more they processed the material, the

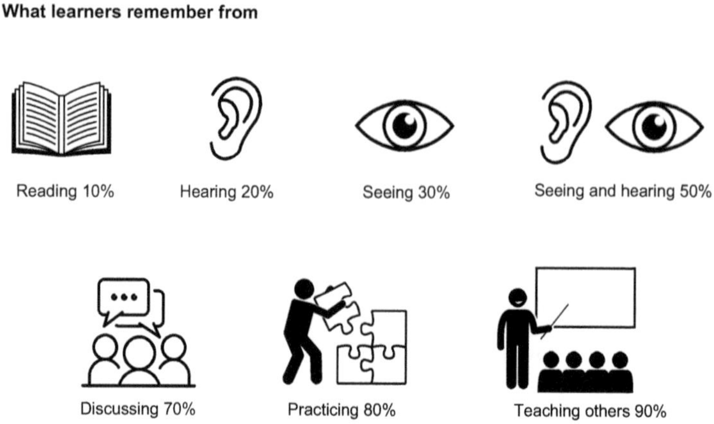

FIGURE 5.2 Memory support.

Illustration created with Canva.

more they remembered, as illustrated in Figure 5.2. Patients often have difficulty remembering and understanding medical information, and 40%–80% of the information provided by healthcare professionals is forgotten immediately. The greater the volume of information delivered, the higher the risk of misunderstanding (Twomey et al., 2020). Supporting patients' memory is therefore crucial to facilitating understanding and helping them manage their situation. Memory is strengthened when learning is relevant, meaningful and actively engaging. Healthcare professionals need to support patients' memory by offering information that is meaningful and relevant to the current situation and by helping them make sense of it, potentially through the use of multiple senses.

How do your patients learn what they need to learn? How do you support their memory?

Support Different Ways of Learning

An important part of the learning process is the individual's approach to learning, which varies from person to person. People have different preferences for how they begin learning something new. Some prefer written or oral information, while others may prefer pictures or videos with explanations. If the purpose is to learn something practical, such as riding a bike, there are also different ways to begin, as described by Kolb (1984) in the model of experiential learning. Some people want to start by watching someone ride a bike. Others prefer to sit on the back while someone else rides and experience what it feels like. Some want to begin by thinking about the principles of riding a bike, and others start by experimenting and working out how it functions.

When healthcare professionals teach patients about self-care, they can ask how the patient prefers to begin learning something new. For example, if the patient is learning to give themselves an injection, they may prefer the healthcare professional first to demonstrate it. The patient can then give themselves an injection under supervision and receive feedback through dialogue with the healthcare professional. Some patients may prefer to prepare in advance. In that case, the healthcare professional can provide written information with pictures or an instructional video, together with an opportunity to ask questions about the content. The patient can then perform the injection with guidance from staff.

> *When you buy a new technical device, what is your preferred way to begin learning about it? Do you read the manual first? Watch someone else use it? Try it while someone guides you. Or start experimenting on your own to work it out?*

Support Reflection

The literature on reflection mainly addresses students' learning through experience in the development of professional competence, particularly in health and medical education (Mann et al., 2009). Boud et al. (1985) describe three aspects of reflection: returning to the experience, attending to feelings and reappraising the experience. The aim is for the learner to explore their understanding of their knowledge and experience, and the effects these have on themselves and others. Kolb (1984) defines learning as a process in which knowledge is created through the transformation of experience. His model of experiential learning includes four phases: concrete experience, observation and reflection, abstract theorising and experimentation. Learning can begin at any phase but proceeds through the four phases in a clockwise direction. In the example above of different ways of learning to ride a bike, the individual's experience is transformed through reflection into a new understanding. If learning begins with observing someone ride a bicycle, the learner starts to reflect on how it is done. This reflection leads to a theoretical understanding of the principles of cycling, and a conclusion can be drawn about how to do it. That understanding is then used in the experimental phase, which produces a new experience to observe and reflect on, such as what worked well, what did not and why. A new theoretical understanding is then constructed about how cycling can be improved, and this is tested in a further experimental phase.

Patients need time to reflect on their experiences and feelings during illness and to relate them to information and instructions they have found or received, so that they can understand themselves and deal with the situation. Reflection can take place individually or together with healthcare professionals, other patients, relatives and others, and it can vary in depth. For some, illness contributes to transformative learning, meaning a changed outlook on life (Mezirow, 2009). Healthcare professionals can support patients in re-evaluating their experiences through critical reflection on their own assumptions, helping them address their situation in a new way. Patients also need time to reflect on all the information they have received so that they can relate it to their own situation, understand it and formulate new questions, including together with relatives. As patients learn and perform different forms of self-care, they observe and reflect on them, and new questions may arise after they return home. If this learning process is not supported, they may experiment in order to find the best way to perform self-care, and errors may occur. It is therefore extremely important, for patients' understanding and management of self-care, that they have access to healthcare professionals after a pedagogical encounter for further questions and concerns.

How do you follow-up patients' understanding? How do you determine whether they have understood the information and instructions, and whether they are able to manage the situation?

Provide Feedback

Feedback is one of the most powerful influences on learning and achievement (Hattie & Timperley, 2007). Researchers in the field have pointed to the need for partnerships between teachers and learners and for shared responsibility in giving and receiving feedback. This aligns with person-centred care, in which partnership between patients and healthcare professionals is essential. Feedback is a dynamic exchange of information between teacher and learner, and it is closely linked to the concept of feedback literacy. Feedback literacy refers to the understandings, capacities and dispositions needed to interpret information and use it to improve work or learning strategies (Carless & Boud,

2018). Feedback is perceived as supportive when it is timely, constructive, delivered by someone trustworthy and accompanied by opportunities to ask questions. However, feedback is more than simply receiving comments from another person. Healthcare students develop internal feedback literacy in clinical practice by comparing thoughts, feelings and behaviours, observing one another, and reflecting on learning experiences (Silén et al., 2025). Teachers and clinical supervisors can support students' learning by encouraging them to reflect on internal feedback.

Patients have reported not understanding the information they receive, which means that healthcare professionals need to assess patients' understanding, skills and competencies and provide feedback accordingly. For feedback to be possible, patients' understanding must be made visible and discussed. Healthcare professionals can ask patients what they have learned from observing others or their surroundings, participating in their own care and reflecting on their experiences. Patients can also be invited to give feedback on the healthcare professional's performance during a pedagogical encounter and to suggest ways of improving communication and support for patient learning. These interactions highlight important skills that healthcare professionals need in order to make care experiences more understandable, manageable and meaningful for patients.

> *How can you invite patients to give you feedback on your performance? How would that feel?*

Practices to Facilitate Patient Learning

A wide range of practices can support clear and meaningful communication in pedagogical encounters with patients. The choice of method should always be guided by the patient's individual needs and abilities, as well as by the healthcare professional's competence, professional judgement and the context of the encounter. Combining several practices – verbal, non-verbal, digital and interactive – can improve understanding and strengthen patient engagement (Kwame & Petrucka, 2021). It is also essential that patient information is accessible, easy to use and designed to minimise misunderstandings. This includes communication methods that accommodate different cognitive or functional abilities, literacy levels and personal preferences. Such considerations align with the Convention on the Rights of Persons with Disabilities (CRPD), which highlights the importance of accessible information for all individuals (United Nations, 2006).

Check Pre-Understanding

Before introducing new information, it is important to explore what the person already knows, understands and is able to do (Hashim, 2017). This helps you adjust both the level of information and the way it is delivered to the patient's needs. Another way to assess pre-understanding is to ask the patient to describe how they handle specific situations, such as taking medication or managing pain. It is also valuable to explore the patient's previous experiences of, and attitudes to, healthcare, illness and treatment, both positive and negative, as well as their current emotional state. Do they have past experiences that influence how they think about healthcare? Are they in an emotional state that allows them to take in, remember and use the information provided? As discussed earlier in this chapter, a patient's emotional state and previous experiences may influence their attention during the encounter and thereby how much information they are able to take in and use. These factors shape both the patient's ability and willingness to understand and retain information during the encounter. Examples of specific questions that can help uncover the patient's pre-understanding, attitudes and emotions are provided in Box 5.1.

BOX 5.1 EXAMPLES OF QUESTIONS TO CHECK PRE-UNDERSTANDING, ATTITUDES AND EMOTIONS

- What do you already know about this condition? Have you heard about it before? Do you know someone who has had it? (comprehensibility)
- What does this condition mean to you personally? How do you feel about it? What concerns or thoughts do you have? (meaningfulness)
- What do you know about the treatment for this condition? Have you heard about any medicines, therapies or other ways to manage it? (comprehensibility)
- How do you usually manage new information or unfamiliar situations? (manageability)
- How do you feel about this right now? Worried, stressed? (meaningfulness)

Use Plain Language

Patients' understanding is supported when healthcare professionals explain things clearly, use plain language and avoid conveying medical jargon. Healthcare professionals often use technical terms and abbreviations that are unfamiliar to patients, which can hinder understanding (Danaher et al., 2023). For example, describing test results as "positive" or "negative" can be confusing because these words have different meanings in everyday language. Instead, state clearly what the result shows, for example, "the test indicates that you have the condition." At the same time, it is important to avoid language that is overly simplified or patronising. Condescending communication, sometimes called "baby talk," can damage trust and reduce patient engagement. The aim should be clear, respectful and supportive communication that preserves dignity and autonomy. Guidance on how to practise Plain Language is presented in Box 5.2.

BOX 5.2 PLAIN LANGUAGE EXERCISE

1. Reflect on the medical jargon, abbreviations and complex words commonly used in health communication in your workplace.
2. Make a list of these terms and identify as many as possible.
3. Go through the list and find alternative words or phrases that are simpler and easier for patients to understand.
4. Reflect on the revised formulations. Are they genuinely easier to understand, or could they still be confusing or misleading for a patient? Ensure that the information uses everyday language that is clear and accessible. If possible, test the revised phrases on different people, including patients, to gather feedback.

Repeat and Focus on Important Information

Repeating a limited number of key messages and reinforcing them increases the likelihood that patients will remember and understand the information. While it may be tempting to convey a large amount of information, doing so can overwhelm patients and reduce retention. To enhance patient understanding and recall:

- Identify the three most important points the patient needs to remember.
- Repeat these points throughout the conversation.

Promote Questions and Information Search

Using questions in a pedagogical encounter supports the patient's attention, processing, motivation and understanding, and provides valuable feedback to both the patient and the healthcare professional. A central goal is to create a situation in which the patient feels comfortable and encouraged to ask questions. This allows them to receive relevant answers, confirm their understanding and ask for clarification. At the same time, the questions patients ask offer insight into how they interpret and understand the information provided.

One way to encourage questions is to use open-ended prompts that cannot be answered with a simple yes or no. Compare how it feels to respond to the following:

1. Have you understood?
2. Do you have any questions?
3. What questions do you have?
4. Which questions would you like to ask?

Closed questions (1 and 2) are easy for patients to dismiss, especially if they feel embarrassed or think there is no time for discussion. Open questions (3 and 4), by contrast, signal that questions are expected and welcome, making it easier for patients to raise concerns.

Another helpful tool is to offer a short list of frequently asked questions (FAQs). Patients may find it difficult to formulate questions in the moment because they feel stressed, are unsure what is appropriate to ask, or simply forget what they intended to say. An FAQ list can help them identify what they want to know. Examples include:

- What do I need to do when I get home?
- For how long should I continue doing this?
- I have heard that . . . is that correct?

A complementary strategy is the Ask Me 3 method (Toibin et al., 2017). It encourages patients to ensure that they receive answers to three essential questions about their health and care. The third question, why, is often overlooked, yet it is crucial because it helps patients understand the meaning behind recommendations and increases their motivation to follow them. The three questions are the following:

- What is my main problem?
- What do I need to do?
- Why is it important for me to do this?

Because patients frequently encounter health information outside the healthcare system, it is also important to encourage them to think critically about the information they find. Questions that explore source credibility can help reveal prior knowledge and support evaluation of the reliability of those sources. These conversations should be handled sensitively so that patients do not feel judged or inadequate. Examples include:

- What do you already know?
- What are your thoughts about this?
- Where did you get that information?

Finally, not all patients know where to find reliable information or possess the digital skills needed to access online resources. Healthcare professionals can support them by recommending trustworthy websites, demonstrating how to navigate them, and, where possible, allowing patients to practise accessing the information during the encounter, for example, on their own phone. Some patients may also have visual or cognitive limitations that make online information difficult to use. In such cases, printed materials, patient associations and patient libraries can provide valuable alternatives. Awareness of these resources enables healthcare professionals to guide patients effectively.

Use Teach-Back

Teach-back is a method used to assess whether a patient has received, understood and interpreted information correctly (Shersher et al., 2021). At the same time, it supports attention, memory, processing and understanding. The method involves selecting the most important information, breaking it into manageable parts and asking the patient to restate those key points in their own words. It is usually better to ask the patient to restate the most important parts one at a time rather than repeat everything at once. Be explicit about what you want the patient to restate, for example, how to take medication or what steps to follow before the next visit. Patients may feel embarrassed or patronised if the request is not phrased carefully. To avoid this, frame the request so that responsibility lies with you as the healthcare professional, rather than implying that the patient has done something wrong. Importantly, teach-back is not only about the patient restating information. It also requires the healthcare professional to restate what the patient has said in order to identify misunderstandings, clarify ambiguities and add information where needed. Examples of prompts for restating are presented in Box 5.3.

BOX 5.3 EXAMPLES OF PROMPTS FOR RESTATING USING TEACH-BACK

- "I know that was a lot of information. Could you tell me in your own words how to take your medicine? That way, I can make sure I explained it clearly."
  . . .[patient retells in their own words]. . .
  "Great, that's correct', or 'thank you, that was quite right. However . . ."
- "We have now talked about why it is important for you to take your medicine. Could you summarise what we talked about?"
  . . .[patient retells in their own words]. . .
  "Great, that's correct', or 'thank you, that was quite right. However . . ."
- "Finally, what would you say you should do if you forget to take it?"
  . . .[patient retells in their own words]. . .
  "Great, that's correct', or 'thank you, that was quite right. However . . ."

Promote Learning by Doing

Actively involving patients in tasks related to their care supports attention, understanding, memory and the ability to apply information in practice. When patients take part in performing tasks themselves, their ability to understand and use health information improves (Lyu et al., 2024). This hands-on involvement also helps strengthen confidence and prepares patients to manage their health. The approach is grounded in principles of active and experiential learning, in which individuals learn by doing, reflecting and applying knowledge in real-life situations (Kolb, 1984). In healthcare, such strategies can support self-management, treatment adherence and the safe performance of self-care tasks.

A practical way to support this is to let patients try out the tasks they have been informed about. This also gives the healthcare professional an opportunity to check whether the patient has understood the information and can apply it correctly. It is also important to allow patients time to reflect on the experience, use internal feedback to make sense of what they did and discuss it together. Questions such as "What worked well?", "What could be done differently?" and "How did it feel to carry out the procedure?" can guide this reflection. Through such dialogue, patients can receive constructive feedback, clarify uncertainties and strengthen their competence and confidence in

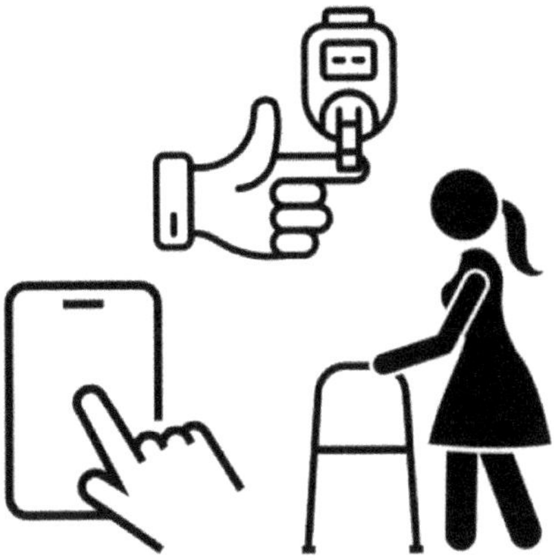

FIGURE 5.3 Examples of learning by doing.

Illustration created with Canva.

managing the task. Examples of learning activities that promote learning by doing (Figure 5.3) include:

- Inviting the patient to log in to a relevant webpage or healthcare app and search for information themselves, rather than only mentioning that the resource exists.
- Demonstrating how to use a walking aid, then asking the patient to show how it should be used.
- Guiding the patient through measuring their own blood pressure or glucose levels and then letting them perform the task independently.

Combine Oral, Written and Language-Adapted Information

Combining written and oral information enhances patients' knowledge, recall and satisfaction (Dima et al., 2026; Johnson et al., 2003). Using several information formats also supports different ways of learning and can reduce cognitive load when patients need to absorb complex or emotionally charged information. Written information may include notes taken during the encounter, either by the healthcare professional or by the patient. Offering paper and a pen can encourage note-taking and help patients feel comfortable doing so. Ready-made patient information materials may also support understanding, but the content must always be relevant to the patient's situation (Menichetti et al., 2021). Relevance is an important condition for meaningful learning, and personalising information can reduce the risk of overload. If parts of the material do not apply, these sections can be crossed out or highlighted to make the information more personal. In addition, adding short, individualised notes can make the information easier to understand and use.

It is also important to recognise that patients differ in how easily they can read and understand written information. Even so, written information may still be useful for those who find reading difficult, for example, if they can share it with relatives or others. Since most patients have mobile phones, it can also be helpful to invite them to record the consultation, as audio or video, if permitted and appropriate, so that they can revisit instructions later, for example, when performing a procedure at home.

Another aspect to consider is language proficiency, which influences how patients receive and process information. When patients are not fluent in the language used in healthcare, understanding information, asking questions and expressing concerns can be particularly challenging. In these situations, a professional interpreter should be used (Jenstad et al., 2024). Although family members may wish to help, they are generally not recommended as interpreters, because this can limit open communication, affect accuracy and make it more difficult to discuss sensitive topics. When working with an interpreter, speak directly to the patient, use clear and simple language and allow time for interpretation. The interpreter's role is to translate exactly what is said, not to simplify, alter or omit content. In addition to spoken communication supported by interpreters, attention should also be given to the quality of written translations. When providing translated written health information, it is essential to ensure that the language is accurate. Migrants sometimes report being cautious about translated materials because of previous experiences with inaccurate translations, and even minor errors can substantially alter the meaning of a text. Translated information should therefore use plain, accessible language rather than academic terminology, and the content should be culturally relevant to the target group.

Use Visual Aids and Augmentative and Alternative Communication

Visual aids, such as videos, images, demonstrations and opportunities to see or handle relevant equipment or tools, can enhance patients' understanding of information and instructions (Galmarini et al., 2024; Schubbe et al., 2020). These methods make information more concrete and easier to remember by linking it to real situations, tools or procedures that patients will encounter in their care. For this reason, visual aids can be useful for many patients and in many situations. Examples of how to use them include:

- Show a needle, IV line or catheter when talking with the patient about these items and explaining that they will be used or inserted.
- Use images or 3D models of the body to illustrate the patient's health condition, explain what is happening inside the body, or demonstrate how it functions.
- Use pictures or models of different foods, accompanied by sugar cubes, to illustrate the amount of sugar each food contains.

One specific type of visual communication is pictorial support, which refers to images designed to enhance written or spoken communication, either alone or combined with short, simple text (Figure 5.4). These can be adapted to different formats depending on the context:

- Communication boards: Multiple images on a single board to facilitate interaction on specific topics, such as reception, consultation or post-surgery care.
- Step-by-step cards: Individual images illustrating stages of a healthcare visit, shown one at a time, arranged on a timeline or placed in a flipbook.
- Integrated images: Pictures alongside text in appointment letters or instructions, reinforcing key actions (e.g. fasting before a visit) and reused during the encounter for consistency.

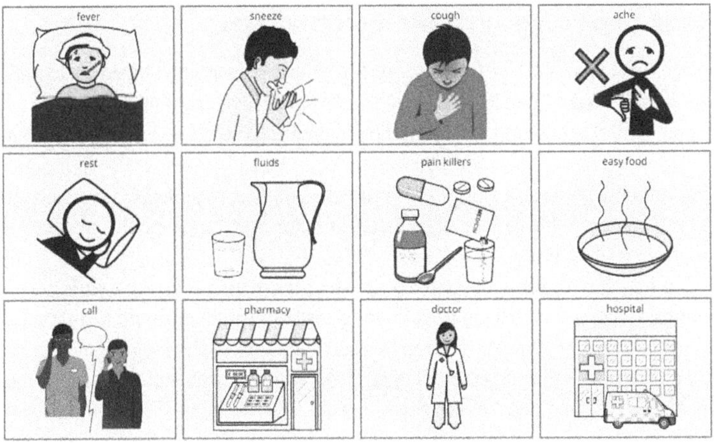

FIGURE 5.4 Pictorial support.

Illustration from www.bildstod.se. For information about the symbols, see vgregion.se/ov/dart/licenser.

When using pictorial support, it is preferable to use specially designed images that have been tested with the specific patient group. Some pictorial supports are accompanied by text showing what is depicted in two languages. If the information is critical, serious or includes important instructions, pictorial support should not replace the use of an interpreter. In general, the following should be kept in mind when using pictorial support:

- If possible, use images that have been tested with your specific target group.
- Point to the images while speaking.
- Place the image centrally and explain how the patient can use it. It is a tool for both healthcare professionals and the patient.
- Allow the patient to ask questions and express themselves using the images.

Augmentative and alternative communication (AAC) includes a broader range of methods designed to support individuals with difficulties in verbal or written expression. These include body-based strategies such as gestures, facial expressions and sign language. Other methods involve tools such as speech-generating devices, AAC apps, eye-tracking systems, picture boards and communication books. While some AAC technologies are intended for individuals with specific communication needs, many simpler AAC tools, including pictorial support, can also facilitate understanding and communication for a wider patient population.

Practising Pedagogical Encounters – Cases

The *Think and Act Patient Learning* framework was developed to explain how theories and concepts related to coping ability, learning and health literacy contribute to understanding how patient learning can be supported during illness. The framework is not intended to be followed literally in practice but rather to serve as a guiding structure that supports healthcare professionals in encounters with patients who need to learn about their health in order to manage it effectively.

In healthcare, some encounters are long-term and recurring, while others are brief and momentary. The following cases illustrate different health situations in different contexts and can be used to practise a pedagogical encounter. The first case, Charlie, is an example of a well-planned and well-conducted pedagogical encounter. In the cases that follow – Kim, Hila and Maria – you can practise applying the framework to identify each patient's individual needs. Each case reveals what capacities and possibilities the patients have for understanding, managing and finding meaning in their current situation, and for learning through the pedagogical encounter.

Illustration Case

Charlie

The first case describes Charlie, an older man whose care history has left him dissatisfied with how his healthcare needs have been managed. In this case, a pedagogical encounter is presented in which the nurse effectively applied the framework.

Charlie, an 80-year-old economics professor, remains intellectually active but has recently stopped writing scientific articles because of Parkinson's disease, diagnosed six years ago. His symptoms – fatigue and bowel and urinary problems – were initially overlooked because he did not have the typical tremors. At present, his vision and hearing are intact, but he has mild cognitive impairment and persistent fatigue, which he feels is not adequately addressed by his care team. He also feels unheard by clinic staff and is saddened by his reduced social life and inability to continue writing. Charlie was treated with dopamine tablets for years, but they lost effectiveness. He was scheduled to try a temporary pump for dopamine administration and had been told to bring the medication himself to the clinic. When he arrived, the procedure was cancelled because he had not understood how to obtain the medication. Charlie felt upset and "objectified" because he had not received clear information beforehand. Eventually the pump was installed and Charlie's symptoms improved – less shaking and fewer bladder and bowel problems – but the fatigue remained. Because he felt that the clinic did not address this fatigue, he decided to try extra dopamine tablets, which made him even more tired. He then considered contacting his doctor but felt too exhausted and discouraged, believing that they would not listen.

At his next appointment, Charlie was told that the extra medication had caused dopamine dysregulation syndrome, but the explanation was difficult to understand because it relied on complex medical terminology. Online searches gave conflicting information, leaving him feeling less in control. He has now been invited to a follow-up appointment with a nurse to review his treatment and discuss surgery for a permanent pump. He is bringing his wife in the hope of getting answers to many questions and finding a sustainable solution to his health problems.

Before the pedagogical encounter, the nurse scheduled a one-hour appointment in a secluded room to ensure that the meeting would not be interrupted. From the medical record, the nurse could see that there had been previous instances of unclear communication that had led to misunderstanding and confusion for the patient. For this reason, the nurse considered it especially important to ground the meeting in a narrative and trust-based relationship. In addition, clear and comprehensive explanations would be crucial to ensure the patient's understanding. The nurse planned to explore the patient's views on his dopamine treatment and find out how motivated he was to proceed with surgery for a permanent pump. By the end of the encounter, the patient and his wife were expected to understand the main benefits of the dopamine pump and have a basic understanding of how the device functions. In addition to verbal information, the nurse prepared written material outlining the pre-operative instructions, along with a brochure describing the dopamine pump and its functions. The nurse also planned to bring a demonstration pump to the meeting.

When planning and conducting the encounter the nurse considered the key aspects of a pedagogical encounter:

Situation: The nurse aimed to create clear, empathetic communication with the patient in order to rebuild his trust and guide him towards safer and more effective management of his treatment.

Agents: The nurse explained her role, expertise and experience in the field. The patient's wife was encouraged to contribute to the conversation and add anything important regarding the patient's needs and situation.

Purpose: The nurse explained that the purpose of the encounter was to discuss the patient's current situation and plan how he could continue his medication using the dopamine pump. The aim was to understand how he felt about his medication, address any questions he had and help him prepare for the upcoming surgery.

Goal: Together with the patient, the nurse identified that he had not fully understood the function of the temporary pump, as he had been taking additional medication to manage his remaining symptoms. The nurse helped him understand that these extra doses did not improve his condition; instead, they increased his fatigue. He acknowledged feeling uncertain about his medication and explained that complex medical terminology, combined with online information-seeking, had not given him the clarity he needed. The nurse wanted to help the patient gain a clear understanding of how his treatment works and of the importance of adhering to a controlled medication regimen. Another goal was that, by the end of the encounter, both the patient and his wife would feel confident in their ability to manage cassette changes independently. The nurse explained that they were not expected to be fully trained on the pump during this visit, as the procedure would be practised in greater detail after surgery.

Intentions: To gain a clear understanding of the current situation, the nurse began by asking the patient about his experience of dopamine treatment and what he already knew about the planned procedure. The nurse then asked about his expectations of the meeting and his future treatment. Through the conversation, the nurse learned that the patient had encountered difficulties in managing his medication and in interpreting and applying health-related information. The nurse also recognised that his health literacy was somewhat limited, which, combined with the effects of his illness, had affected his ability to manage care effectively. Despite these challenges, the nurse noted that he was a well-educated man with a strong socio-economic background and a generally high, though currently unstable, SOC.

Interaction: The nurse asked the patient about his current situation, as well as his own perceptions and pre-understanding. The presence of the patient's wife was important because she could help him remember the questions he wanted to ask and later remind him of what had been discussed during the encounter. The nurse also encouraged the patient's wife to join the conversation, ask questions and confirm their understanding by restating the information in their own words. The nurse first provided the necessary information and then, to confirm his understanding, asked him to repeat it back, allowing time for questions throughout.

Content: The basic functions of the pump were introduced, and the nurse explained that the medication cassette would need to be replaced weekly. The nurse also provided written and verbal information about the pre-operative preparations. Given the patient's mild cognitive decline and fatigue, the nurse communicated clearly and avoided complex medical terminology.

Activities: The nurse provided both instruction and a hands-on demonstration of how to change the dopamine cassette, ensuring that the patient and his wife had enough time to reflect and ask questions. At this stage, the goal was simply to familiarise them with the pump and the medication cassette; a more detailed demonstration and practice would be needed after surgery. The nurse also gave detailed information about whom to contact at the clinic if needed.

After the pedagogical encounter, the nurse asked the patient and his wife for feedback on any uncertainties regarding the meeting, thereby fostering a collaborative and supportive environment. Follow-up of what the patient had learned during the encounter showed that he understood how the treatment worked and what his own role was in managing it. He also gained insight into the cause of his fatigue and how he might cope with it. This strengthened his motivation to continue treatment using the implanted automatic pump and to learn how to manage the associated self-care tasks. He felt that the physician and nurse listened to him and understood his concerns, which contributed to a sense of trust and to feeling treated with respect.

Cases for Practice

The following three cases are designed to encourage you and your team to reflect on, and discuss, how patient learning can be effectively facilitated. When planning and conducting pedagogical encounters in these cases, it is essential to consider the learning environment, teaching approaches and the use of clear and meaningful communication to support the learning process when applying the model for creating a pedagogical encounter. You can use Table 5.1 when discussing these cases.

Kim

Kim is a 56-year-old construction worker with no previous history of illness or chronic disease. While working onsite, a small iron beam accidentally fell on his shin, causing a wound. A nurse at his workplace applied a basic dressing and advised him to monitor the injury himself. After a few days, Kim noticed that the wound had developed a foul odour and was leaking a thick yellow fluid. Concerned, he returned to the nurse, who replaced the dressing and recommended that he contact his primary care physician. However, Kim found this difficult: accessing care required navigating an online system, and he was unsure where to begin.

Feeling uncertain, Kim turned to the internet to search for information about his symptoms, where he encountered conflicting and non-specific advice. This increased his uncertainty, and he was unable to determine whether the information applied to his situation. Because the wound was not painful, he underestimated its seriousness and began to lose motivation to seek further care, assuming that it might heal with time. Several more days passed and the wound continued to worsen. Eventually, Kim's wife stepped in to help him identify the appropriate primary care centre. Upon contacting the clinic, Kim was placed on a waiting list and instructed first to provide blood samples. He was then asked to contact the clinic again once the results were available, further delaying direct medical intervention. Another week passed, and Kim remained unaware that he was expected to check his test results online. Meanwhile, his condition deteriorated: his leg began to hurt and he developed a fever. With growing concern, he sought emergency care for the wound. Upon arrival, Kim was visibly frustrated and confused, struggling to understand how the situation had escalated despite his efforts to follow instructions.

Questions to reflect on when you use this case for practice:

- If you were working in the emergency department that day, how would you conduct the pedagogical encounter with Kim?
- What are your thoughts on his own health resources and abilities with regard to SOC and health literacy?

- How would you assess Kim's situation, and how could you help him feel more comfortable?
- What is essential for Kim to understand and do after this encounter?
- How can you specifically support his learning process?
- How can you follow up Kim's understanding?
- What challenges might Kim face in future when managing his own care and navigating the healthcare system? Is there anything you can do at this stage to prepare him for that?

Hila

Hila is a 35-year-old woman who migrated to her current country of residence about seven years ago. She has always been interested in learning new things, but she only had the opportunity to attend school for a few years. She learned to read and do basic mathematics, but has had little opportunity to practise these skills since then, as she has spent most of her adult life working at home and on the farm. When she arrived in Sweden, she began a beginner's Swedish course but had to drop out when her first child was born. She never resumed her studies, as she had several children in quick succession, leaving her with no time for education. She now spends her days at home and in her neighbourhood. Apart from her family, she occasionally meets some neighbours who share her native language.

Hila has been feeling tired for a long time and has started to find it troublesome constantly to need to urinate. She has explained this to herself by thinking that one of her four children, aged three to seven, always wakes her at night and that she has started drinking a great deal of coffee and soft drinks to stay awake. One of her neighbours, to whom she confided her problems, pointed out that these could also be symptoms of diabetes, which eventually led her to contact healthcare services by phone.

During the first visit, she was able to describe her symptoms and have some tests taken. An interpreter was present to facilitate communication between her and the healthcare staff. Despite this, she found it difficult to understand what was being said. On a few occasions, she was asked whether she understood, but instead of admitting that she did not, she nodded. She felt that she ought to understand and did not want to appear unintelligent. A week later, she received a letter from the healthcare provider with an appointment for a follow-up visit. To understand the content, she asked a neighbour to help her read and translate the letter. However, Hila was not entirely sure that the neighbour had translated everything correctly but had to rely on her because she could not understand a single word herself.

The following week, she visited the healthcare centre again, but unfortunately on the wrong day and at the wrong time, because the neighbour had misunderstood that part of the information. As a result, she received a bill for a missed appointment and a new appointment, this time communicated to her verbally by the receptionist. She is now sitting in the waiting room and is about to meet the doctor, who, based on her previous visit and test results, has concluded that she has type 2 diabetes.

Questions to reflect on when you use this case for practice:

- What are your intentions and approaches for the encounter?
- How would you appraise Hila's situation, and what can you do to help her feel more at ease?
- What are your thoughts on her health resources and abilities with regard to SOC and health literacy?
- What is Hila expected to understand at the end of the encounter?
- What does she need to learn to take responsibility for her own care, well-being and health? How can you specifically support her learning process?
- How can you follow up Hila's understanding?
- What challenges do you foresee for Hila in managing her new life situation?

Maria

Maria is a 65-year-old full-time teacher who has been experiencing persistent headaches for several months. To understand the cause of her symptoms, she initially tried to manage the situation on her own by reading about different types of headaches and consulting a physiotherapist. Despite these efforts, her symptoms continued without improvement, which led her to contact her general practitioner. Because of a long waiting list at the clinic, Maria was offered only a brief telephone appointment instead of the in-person visit she had hoped for. This left her feeling frustrated, as she had expected a longer consultation in which she would have an opportunity to discuss her situation in depth.

When the telephone appointment eventually took place, the doctor informed her that he had only five minutes available. Maria found this limited timeframe insufficient to describe her symptoms properly. She also felt that some of the questions asked were irrelevant and consumed valuable time.

In addition, she felt that the doctor interrupted her attempts to explain her concerns, which contributed to a growing sense of confusion and mistrust. The call ended with the doctor stating that he would order blood tests and that Maria could schedule a follow-up appointment at the clinic. Although she appreciated that further steps were being taken, the overall experience left her feeling unheard and uncertain whether her concerns were being taken seriously.

> Questions to reflect on when you use this case for practice:
>
> - If you were that doctor, how would you spend those five minutes of the telephone consultation to ensure that relevant information was obtained, and trust was built with the patient?
> - Think about which questions you could ask to narrow down the information you need about the patient's understanding, expectations and motivation.
> - How could you help her feel more comfortable and seen?
> - How can you follow up on Maria's understanding?

Concluding Remarks on the Cases

The cases presented in this chapter illustrate different prerequisites for learning during illness, and how the model for a pedagogical encounter can be applied in different ways. What they all share, however, is that conducting such a meeting early in the patient's learning process can be highly beneficial.

In Charlie's case, numerous learning difficulties arose because of unclear communication from healthcare professionals and conflicting online information, all of which contributed to a reduced sense of control over his care. A pedagogical encounter early in his treatment journey would likely have prevented much of this confusion.

For Kim, a pedagogical encounter in the emergency department would reveal his limited ability to navigate online systems and interpret conflicting digital information. This shared understanding would enable healthcare professionals to guide him towards reliable sources of information and appropriate healthcare contact points.

In Hila's case, despite the presence of an interpreter, she did not fully understand what was communicated during her initial visit with the doctor. A pedagogical encounter where the doctor actively ensured her understanding, could have helped identify her difficulties at an early stage, enabling timely support and promoting safe, person-centred care.

In Maria's case, the limited time available for the appointment is the primary challenge, which underscores the importance of being well prepared to support her learning. When used thoughtfully, even a brief encounter can be meaningful and help her feel seen, taken seriously and genuinely cared for.

Summary

Pedagogical competence among healthcare professionals is crucial for supporting patients' learning, self-care, health and well-being. The *Think and Act Patient Learning* framework is aligned with person-centred care and aims to help healthcare professionals facilitate each individual patient's learning process. A trusting relationship is a prerequisite and can be established through a pedagogical encounter. Thinking in terms of patient learning is grounded in theory and research on sense of coherence, learning during illness, and health literacy. Acting in terms of patient learning means creating a pedagogical encounter and facilitating learning by using approaches and practices that make learning possible. In Chapter 6, the prerequisites for implementing pedagogical competence development for healthcare students and professionals within healthcare organisations will be discussed.

References

Biggs, J., & Tang, C. (2011). *Teaching for quality learning at university* (4th ed.). Society for Research into Higher Education & Open University Press.

Boman, E. L., Sandelin, K., Wengström, Y., & Silén, C. (2018). Patients' participation during treatment and care of breast cancer – a possibility and an imperative. *European Journal of Oncology Nursing*, 37, 35–42. https://doi.org/10.1016/j.ejon.2018.09.002

Boud, D., Keogh, R., & Walker, D. (1985). *Reflection: Turning experience into learning*. Kogan Page.

Carless, D., & Boud, D. (2018). The development of student feedback literacy: Enabling uptake of feedback. *Assessment & Evaluation in Higher Education*, 43(8), 1315–1325. https://doi.org/10.1080/02602938.2018.1463354

Danaher, T. S., Author, A. A., Author, B. B., & Author, C. C. (2023). Improving how clinicians communicate with patients: An integrative review and framework. *Journal of Service Research*, 26(4), 493–510. https://doi.org/10.1177/10946705231190018

Dima, D. C., Sium, A., Giuliani, M., & Papadakos, J. (2026). Enduring power of print: How health information pamphlets promote equity and trust in patient education. *JCO Oncology Practice*, 22(4), 555–558. https://doi.org/10.1200/OP-25-00739

Eriksen, A. A., Fegran, L., Fredwall, T. E., & Larsen, I. B. (2023). Patients' negative experiences with health care settings brought to light by formal complaints: A qualitative metasynthesis. *Journal of Clinical Nursing*. https://doi.org/10.1111/jocn.16704

Galmarini, E., Marciano, L., & Schulz, P. J. (2024). The effectiveness of visual-based interventions on health literacy in health care: A systematic review and meta-analysis. *BMC Health Services Research*, 24, 718. https://doi.org/10.1186/s12913-024-11138-1

Hashim, M. J. (2017). Patient-centered communication: Basic skills. *American Family Physician*, 95(1), 29–34.

Hattie, J. T., & Timperley, H. (2007). The power of feedback. *Review of Educational Research*, 77(1), 81–112. https://doi.org/10.3102/003465430298487

Illeris, K. (Ed.). (2009). *Contemporary theories of learning: Learning theorists . . . in their own words* (1st ed.). Routledge. https://doi.org/10.4324/9780203870426

Jenstad, L. M., Howe, T., Breau, G., Abel, J., Colozzo, P., Halas, G., Mason, G., Rieger, C., Simon, L., & Strachan, S. (2024). Communication between healthcare providers and communicatively-vulnerable patients with associated health outcomes: A scoping review of knowledge syntheses. *Patient Education and Counseling*, 119, 108040. https://doi.org/10.1016/j.pec.2023.108040

Johnson, A., Sandford, J., & Tyndall, J. (2003). Written and verbal information versus verbal information only for patients being discharged from acute hospital settings to home. *Cochrane Database of Systematic Reviews*, 2003(4), CD003716. https://doi.org/10.1002/14651858.CD003716

Kolb, D. A. (1984). *Experiential learning*. Prentice Hall.

Kwame, A., & Petrucka, P. M. (2021). A literature-based study of patient-centered care and communication in nurse-patient interactions: Barriers, facilitators, and the way forward. *BMC Nursing*, 20(158). https://doi.org/10.1186/s12912-021-00684-2

Lyu, X., Li, J., & Li, S. (2024). Approaches to reach trustworthy patient education: A narrative review. *Healthcare*, 12(23), 2322. https://doi.org/10.3390/healthcare12232322

Mann, K., Gordon, J., & MacLeod, A. (2009). Reflection and reflective practice in health professions education: A systematic review. *Advances in Health Sciences Education*, 14, 595–621. https://doi.org/10.1007/s10459-007-9090-2

Menichetti, J., Lie, H. C., Mellblom, A. V., Brembo, E. A., Eide, H., Gulbrandsen, P., Heyn, L., Saltveit, K. H., Strømme, H., Sundling, V., Turk, E., & Juvet, L. K. (2021). Tested communication strategies for providing information to patients in medical consultations: A scoping review and quality assessment of the literature. *Patient Education and Counseling*, 104(8), 1891–1903. https://doi.org/10.1016/j.pec.2021.01.019

Mezirow, J. (2009). An overview on transformative learning. In K. Illeris (Ed.), *Contemporary theories of learning: Learning theorists in their own words* (1st ed., pp. 90–105). Routledge.

Nye, C. M., Tengelin, E., & Somayaji, D. (2023). Developing a theory of norm-criticism in nursing education. *Advances in Nursing Science*, 46(2), E66–E79. https://doi.org/10.1097/ANS.0000000000000440

Orem, D. E. (2001). *Nursing: Concepts of practice* (6th ed.). Mosby.
Ramsden, P. (2003). *Learning to teach in higher education* (2nd ed.). Routledge Falmer.
Rusticus, S. A., Pashootan, T., & Mah, A. (2023). What are the key elements of a positive learning environment? Perspectives from students and faculty. *Learning Environments Research*, 26, 161–175. https://doi.org/10.1007/s10984-022-09410-4
Schubbe, D., Scalia, P., Yen, R. W., Saunders, C. H., Cohen, S., Elwyn, G., van den Muijsenbergh, M., & Durand, M.-A. (2020). Using pictures to convey health information: A systematic review and meta-analysis of the effects on patient and consumer health behaviors and outcomes. *Patient Education and Counseling*, 103(10), 1935–1960. https://doi.org/10.1016/j.pec.2020.04.010
Shersher, V., Haines, T. P., Sturgiss, L., Weller, C., & Williams, C. (2021). Definitions and use of the teach-back method in healthcare consultations with patients: A systematic review and thematic synthesis. *Patient Education and Counseling*, 104(1), 118–129. https://doi.org/10.1016/j.pec.2020.07.026
Silén, C. (2013). Learning in the medicine and health care field (Lärande inom medicin och vårdområdet). In C. Silén & K. Bolander Laksov (Eds.), *Creating pedagogical encounters in medicin and healthcare* (*Att Skapa pedagogiska Möten i medicin och vård*). Studentlitteratur.
Silén, C., Kilström, D., & Karlgren, K. (2025). Discerning and acknowledging diverse types of feedback in clinical practice – a way to develop feedback literacy. *Assessment & Evaluation in Higher Education*, 50(1), 159–171. https://doi.org/10.1080/02602938.2024.2369604
Toibin, M., Pender, M., & Cusack, T. (2017). The effect of a healthcare communication intervention – ask me 3; on health literacy and participation in patients attending physiotherapy. *European Journal of Physiotherapy*, 19(sup1), 12–14. https://doi.org/10.1080/21679169.2017.1381318
Twomey, M., Sammon, D., & Nagle, T. (2020). Memory recall/information retrieval challenges within the medical appointment: A review of the literature. *Journal of Decision Systems*, 29(3), 148–181. https://doi.org/10.1080/12460125.2020.1809
United Nations. (2006). *Convention on the rights of persons with disabilities*. https://www.un.org/development/desa/disabilities/convention-on-the-rights-of-persons-with-disabilities.html

6

REFLECTIONS ON IMPLEMENTING THE THINK AND ACT PATIENT LEARNING FRAMEWORK

Lena Engqvist Boman, Ann Langius-Eklöf, Kay Sundberg and Josefin Wångdahl

> *Have you ever tried to improve patient care in a structured way, only to find that implementing your ideas either went very well, did not go as planned or worked temporarily but ultimately wasn't sustainable? What do you think were the key factors behind both the successes and the challenges? If you had the chance to do it again, what would you approach differently?*

Implementing new practices in a workplace is a challenging and complex process. It involves many individuals and requires knowledge, skills, time, resources, commitment, support and acceptance within an organisation. While implementation depends heavily on policy, societal and organisational contexts, it also requires practical structures and support across these levels to succeed. This chapter discusses the macro, meso and micro levels of context within healthcare on which the implementation of the *Think and Act Patient Learning* framework depends. It highlights the influence of policy, person-centredness and digitalisation in healthcare, and presents examples of implementing the framework in different healthcare contexts. Although the engagement of individual healthcare professionals is valuable, sustainable implementation requires systems that enable and reinforce these practices. Patient learning is an individual process, yet it also requires prerequisites at all levels to be successfully achieved.

Impact of Contextual Factors

All learning, including learning during illness, occurs in context-dependent situations. Implementation of the framework is influenced by the broader

DOI: 10.4324/9781003540861-7

context across macro, meso and micro levels. At the macro level, national policies, societal structures, norms, values, beliefs and resources shape how healthcare organisations can fulfil their missions. At the meso level, these organisations play an important role in providing training, support and opportunities for healthcare professionals and students to develop their competences. The micro level concerns the units in which the intervention is implemented and includes management support for staff and their individual knowledge, skills and approaches to supporting patient learning. Experts in the field highlight the dynamic nature of context, including the relationship between context, the intervention and its implementation, as well as the interplay among the factors that shape context (Bate, 2014). One review of how context influences successful quality improvement in healthcare showed that most studies focused on one level rather than on the interaction among levels (Fulop & Robert, 2015). Macro contexts, such as health systems, are usually too large and distant to be managed by healthcare professionals, compared with meso organisational contexts or micro team contexts. Policies, laws and regulations at the macro level must therefore legitimise and enable ways of working that promote and support implementation. These structural and regulatory foundations are essential if improvement efforts are not to become isolated, unsustainable or short-lived.

At the meso level, organisational leadership, culture, capacity and the availability of technical infrastructure interact with individual skills, readiness for change and the quality of interpersonal relationships at the micro level. Both large-scale, long-term implementation and smaller, short-term initiatives require structures at all levels that actively and systematically support patients' health and well-being. Without clear organisational support, professionals often lack the time, mandate and resources needed to integrate quality improvements such as the *Think and Act Patient Learning* framework into everyday practice. The requirements for patient learning at the micro level were addressed in earlier chapters, which focused on how patients learn and manage illness and on how healthcare professionals can best support this process.

Policies and Person-Centredness

In many Western countries, laws and policies state that patients should be partners in relation to disease or threat thereof. Central to this is the right to be informed and involved in decisions, as formulated, for example, by the National Institute for Health and Care Excellence in the UK, the National Institutes of Health in the USA, and by legislation in Sweden. In countries where this is not explicitly addressed in laws or official recommendations, other recommendations often indirectly support patient participation at both individual and organisational levels. These may include guidance that information should be accessible and understandable, and that patients should be involved in decisions concerning treatment and health. Several such policies and recommendations emphasise a person-centred care perspective. These structures also contain power relations that may affect healthcare professionals' ability to design and implement interventions aimed at improving patient health and well-being (Ocloo et al., 2020). In addition, an inherent power imbalance exists because of healthcare professionals' authority and patients' vulnerability.

Person-centred care in healthcare involves integrating the patient as an active member of the care team, grounded in the patient's values, preferences, engagement and support needs, together with the competence of healthcare professionals (McCormack et al., 2021). This relies on mutual trust and confidence between patients and professionals. However, implementing person-centred care requires an organisational context that promotes shared decision-making and ensures that healthcare professionals possess the necessary competence. Outcomes such as patient satisfaction, participation, well-being and perceptions of the therapeutic environment must also be evaluated continuously to assess effectiveness and identify areas for improvement.

Studies report positive effects of implementing person-centred care, but few such effects are sustained over time, which underscores the importance of adopting a salutogenic perspective to achieve the best possible outcomes (Ehk et al., 2024). One reason may be that person-centred care is not implemented in line with its definition throughout the organisation (Ekman et al., 2021). Responsibility for enabling professionals to implement person-centred care lies with the organisation, whether at the level of a hospital, primary healthcare centre or smaller unit. It is therefore important that organisations maintain a balance between salutogenic and biomedical perspectives on health. Focus should extend beyond identifying patients' risk factors to include factors that promote health. Healthcare organisations bear ultimate responsibility for the quality of care, for systematic evaluation of processes, and for safeguarding care activities. To realise the policies that govern healthcare, professionals must act as active partners and advocates for patients as participating members of the care team, while promoting thinking and acting patient learning. At the same time, participation in the care team can take different forms, as patients vary in how involved they wish to be. Some may want to be highly active in decision-making, whereas others may prefer a more passive role and want professionals to decide on their behalf. Preferences for participation in treatment and care decisions depend on patients' understanding, abilities, and needs in a specific situation. Respectful treatment by healthcare staff contributes to a sense of being "seen" as a human being, which forms a basis for patient participation (Boman et al., 2018).

World Health Organization Regional Office for Europe (2023) has published a guide on therapeutic patient education, an intervention shown to improve outcomes and quality of life for people living with chronic diseases. The guide offers practical advice to decision-makers at the macro level and to healthcare professionals at the meso level on how to develop and implement such education at the micro level. The purpose of therapeutic patient education is to support a person-centred learning process for people with chronic conditions such as diabetes, high blood pressure and respiratory diseases, so that they can manage self-care, well-being and quality of life. The goal is to increase patients' knowledge, skills and confidence in changing behaviour and in self-managing their condition. Therapeutic patient education is not simple information transfer but a complex, person-centred process grounded in adult learning principles and health literacy. This education can be delivered through information sharing and skills training during a clinical visit, in an inpatient setting, by telephone, or online. The guide emphasises that support for learning should form part of routine care for patients with chronic diseases. This aligns with the *Think and Act Patient Learning* framework, which emphasises continuous support through a person-centred learning process. Grounded in a salutogenic approach, a health-promoting perspective adds to understanding of the patient's learning process during illness as conceptualised through sense of coherence (SOC) and health literacy. These perspectives underpin all pedagogical encounters in healthcare, whether in structured and carefully planned settings or in more spontaneous, improvised situations.

Supporting patient learning at the micro level requires person-centred care to be integrated into the healthcare system at meso and macro levels as well. The need to adopt a health literacy perspective is increasingly recognised in international and national laws, guidelines and public health strategies as essential to ensuring person-centred, safe and equitable care; enabling effective use of healthcare services; and promoting health and sustainability (M-POHL, 2023; Sørensen et al., 2021). These policies typically aim to improve both individual and organisational health literacy and to equip healthcare professionals with the skills needed to support patients' understanding, engagement and participation in care.

A health-literate organisation refers to the degree to which an organisation equitably enables individuals to access, understand and use information and services appropriately in order to make health-related decisions and take action for themselves and others (Centers for Disease Control and Prevention, 2023). The importance of integrating this approach across all levels of healthcare systems is widely emphasised, together with strategies and methods that support clear communication between caregivers and patients in pedagogical encounters (Farmanova et al., 2018). One strategy that operationalises what it means to be a health-literate healthcare organisation is the Ten Attributes of a Health Literate Organization (Brach et al., 2012). These attributes highlight that a health-literate organisation ensures that patients receive accessible, understandable and actionable information and services, which are fundamental conditions for supporting patient learning (Box 6.1).

BOX 6.1 THE TEN ATTRIBUTES OF A HEALTH LITERATE ORGANIZATION (BRACH ET AL., 2012)

1. Has leadership that makes health literacy integral to its mission, structure and operations.
2. Integrates health literacy into planning, evaluation, patient safety, quality improvement.
3. Prepares the workforce to be health literate and monitors progress.
4. Includes populations served in the design, implementation and evaluation of health information and services.
5. Meets the needs of populations with a range of health literacy skills and avoids stigmatisation.
6. Uses health literacy strategies in interpersonal communications and confirms understanding at all points of contact.
7. Provides easy access to health information and services and navigation assistance.
8. Designs/distributes print, audiovisual, social media content which are easy to understand and act on.
9. Addresses health literacy in high-risk situations, including care transitions and communications about medicines.
10. Communicates clearly what health plans cover and what individuals will have to pay for services.

Central to the ten attributes is strong leadership commitment, with health literacy integrated into the organisation's mission, policies, planning and daily operations. Such commitment includes allocating resources for staff training and adapting organisational structures to create the conditions in which patient-learning supportive methods can be implemented. The attributes also stress that staff must be prepared to support individuals with varying levels of health literacy, and that informational materials and care interventions should be adapted accordingly. A healthcare environment, whether physical or digital, that is easy to navigate, with clear displays and user-friendly digital interfaces, also supports patient learning by reducing unnecessary barriers. Universal design principles help ensure that information is accessible and comprehensible for all patients, regardless of language, literacy level, or physical, sensory, or cognitive differences. Moreover, a health-literate organisation actively involves patients and relatives in shaping strategies that strengthen their ability to access, understand, appraise and apply health information, thereby directly fostering meaningful and sustainable patient learning.

Digitalisation of Healthcare Supporting Patient Learning

WHO (2021) defines digital health as an umbrella term encompassing eHealth, the use of digital technologies such as electronic health records and online services, and mHealth, health practices supported by mobile devices such as smartphones and monitoring tools. The digitalisation of healthcare to enhance and support self-care has expanded and now strongly influences physical encounters between healthcare professionals and patients. A wide range of digital systems is available, from booking appointments and accessing medical records to tools that provide education, self-care strategies and symptom monitoring. These tools can offer medication reminders and support tracking of physical activity, blood pressure or blood glucose levels, to name only a few examples. In addition, patients have access to a vast amount of health-related information on the internet. On the one hand, these tools may allow rapid and flexible exchange of information about a person's health and well-being. On the other hand, they are often not connected to immediate feedback from healthcare professionals. Some are evidence-based and developed thoroughly with experts, but many are not and may contain misleading inaccuracies.

In healthcare today, electronic patient-reported outcomes (ePRO) are commonly used to support self-care. Although there are indications that this can facilitate person-centred care, best outcomes seem to be achieved when it is combined with feedback from healthcare professionals (Hang et al., 2024). Digitalisation therefore does not replace the pedagogical encounter but adds new dimensions to it, requiring healthcare professionals to integrate digital tools with person-centred communication. One example from a research project involving patients with cancer during and after treatment is an app based on the SOC concept to facilitate person-centred care, developed to support pedagogical encounters in clinical care (Langius-Eklöf et al., 2017, 2025). The app was designed with awareness that patients manage health situations in different ways and focused on strengthening comprehensibility, manageability and meaningfulness according to individual needs and preferences. It consisted of the following components: (1) a questionnaire allowing patients to assess the occurrence, frequency and distress of symptoms and concerns, available in real time to healthcare providers, (2) a space for free-text comments about other thoughts or concerns, (3) a risk-assessment model for symptoms of concern that sent text-message alerts to healthcare providers, (4) continuous access to evidence-based self-care advice related to reported symptoms and links to relevant websites for further information, (5) graphs enabling patients and healthcare providers to view the history of symptom reporting.

Symptom alerts initiated interaction between nurse and patient, with telephone contact used to discuss reported problems. Pedagogical encounters with a nurse based on the reports were then scheduled in agreement with the patient. The intervention has been scientifically evaluated in more than 20 publications, showing that the app functioned as a supportive tool for patients and nurses in pedagogical encounters and led to reduced symptom burden, higher quality-adjusted life years (QALY) and higher health literacy. Adherence to symptom reporting as intended was high, whereas use of the other app components varied across individuals. Some patients consistently engaged with the self-care advice, graphs or free-text functions, whereas others used these features less frequently. In interviews, patients reported feeling safe and secure when using the app and stated that it facilitated person-centred contact with healthcare professionals. Nurses perceived that the reports generated by the app supported the pedagogical encounter by enabling easier identification of patients' support needs and more focused feedback. They also believed that, for this routine to be well received in standard care, organisations and managers needed sufficient preparedness when implementing digital technologies. Challenges such as time constraints, varying digital skills and workflow integration must therefore be addressed. Organisational readiness and competence development among healthcare professionals are thus crucial when introducing new digital routines.

It is important to acknowledge that, although research demonstrates several advantages of digital tools for self-care, such as facilitating patient empowerment and personalisation, multiple factors influence their actual use (Madanian et al., 2023; Keeling et al., 2025). Barriers include patients' levels of digital health literacy and general health literacy, concerns about personal integrity, professionals' scepticism, technological challenges such as data safety and ownership, and costs and lack of overall guidelines. People with greater health needs and language barriers still struggle to use digital health services and technologies, mainly because of limited access, poor adaptation of services to diverse needs and inequalities in digital infrastructure across Europe (World Health Organization Regional Office for Europe, 2022). Moreover, the use of digital tools to support self-care presupposes internet access and patients' knowledge and skills in navigating the rapidly expanding digital landscape in healthcare.

In present and future pedagogical encounters, the focus will not only be on providing information but also on guiding patients through information they have obtained themselves. Supporting patients in assessing the reliability of digital sources is therefore becoming an increasingly important pedagogical task.

Societal Organisations Supporting Patient Learning

Patients often spend only a short time in the healthcare system, yet their need for support may arise between visits and continue long after treatment. In many countries, patients can receive support in learning and managing their situation from organisations outside the healthcare system. These organisations may be initiated by healthcare professionals, patients, relatives or nonprofit associations. Funding comes from various sources, including private funds, membership fees, healthcare organisations and the business community. Many are run by volunteers, including patients and healthcare professionals (Doble et al., 2024). Patient associations and peer groups are important complements to healthcare support for patient learning and disease management. Patients, caregivers and trained peer mentors have highlighted the unique value of sharing experiences of living with and managing chronic illness, even within an uncertain future (Elliott et al., 2022). However, support groups do not suit everyone and may also cause stress, especially if patients feel overwhelmed by unwanted information or reactions (Palant & Himmel, 2019).

The European Patients Forum website presents different types of patient organisations at local, regional, European and international levels. Some groups support patients with different diagnoses, whereas others focus on people with similar illnesses. Two examples of social support are presented below to illustrate the advantages and disadvantages of different approaches. The first was initiated by patients with cancer in Sweden. The second concerns support for patients with chronic diseases in Norway and was launched by national authorities.

A meeting place for patients diagnosed with cancer and their relatives, Kraftens hus, was established in Sweden and is available at five physical locations as well as online (kraftenshus.se). Its goal is to support patients with cancer and their families in managing their new situation. Anyone who has or has had cancer, or is a relative of someone who has or has died from cancer, is welcome. Visitors can receive emotional, social and practical support, as well as increased knowledge. They can share thoughts, feelings and experiences with others affected by cancer in a safe community and gain concrete tools to navigate a changed life more effectively.

The initiative for Kraftens hus came from people affected by cancer at the micro level, and the organisation has been developed through collaboration among them, the public sector, business, academia and civil society at the meso level. The strongest need among those affected by cancer was to meet others in the same situation in an informal setting and share experiences. In addition to a drop-in café concept, several activities are offered each week. These are based on visitors' needs and wishes and may include lectures, discussion groups, painting or writing and physical activities such as dancing, walking and yoga. In an evaluation, visitors to Kraftens hus reported gaining knowledge and experiences that contributed to stronger self-esteem, greater capacity for self-care and better functioning in daily life (Smith et al., 2021). Kraftens hus also collaborates with researchers to study how knowledgeable patients and relatives can serve as a resource in healthcare development. The model has been successfully developed and implemented in different parts of the country. However, the question remains of who should bear primary responsibility for funding.

Læring og mestringsentre (Learning and Mastery Centres) were established in Norway in 1997 as a statutory part of the Norwegian health and care service to support patients with chronic illnesses and their relatives. Today, these centres are integrated into health and care activities across Norway, from health promotion and prevention to rehabilitation and palliative care (mestring.no). Patients and relatives are offered educational activities intended to strengthen health skills, disease management and quality of life. Learning objectives depend on the target group and range from acquiring sufficient information about an issue to managing complex health challenges. Educational activities include information, teaching, supervision, advice and exchange of experiences, both individually and in groups. Pedagogical principles and tools that promote learning, manageability and health, referred to as health pedagogy, form the basis of education designed collaboratively by healthcare professionals, patients and relatives. These activities take place in specialist and municipal healthcare and in the voluntary sector. The National Competence Service for Learning and Mastery in Healthcare supports the centres nationally through competence development and research.

A study of one Learning and Mastery Centre showed that, although the aim was to create courses collaboratively among patients, relatives and healthcare professionals, user participation was practised as "being involved" rather than "having influence" (Førland, 2014). To increase user influence on course development, it was proposed that healthcare professionals should receive support regarding learning perspectives, salutogenesis and health literacy. The sustainable implementation of the Learning and Mastery Centres can be explained by requirements from Norwegian authorities at the macro level and by national support for competence development and research. The centres are integrated into the publicly financed Norwegian healthcare system. To fulfil the aims of the centres at the meso level, follow-up of how users perceive their participation is needed, and healthcare professionals require competence development in learning, health promotion, salutogenesis and health literacy at the micro level (Førland, 2014). This aligns with the *Think and Act Patient Learning* framework presented in this book.

Competence Development in Thinking and Acting Patient Learning

An important part of implementing the framework is training healthcare professionals in the principles and practice of supporting patient learning. All healthcare professionals can benefit from continuous competence development, supported by policymakers introducing mandatory courses in patient learning for undergraduate students in health and medical education. This foundation can then be strengthened through further education after graduation as part of continuing professional development. Where possible, interprofessional education is beneficial, with all members of a team or work group trained together. To use the *Think and Act Patient Learning* framework, staff need to understand what it means to adopt a salutogenic approach and to support patients' SOC, learning during illness and health literacy in the pedagogical encounter. To illustrate how the use of the framework can be beneficial for competence development, some examples are given below. The pedagogy is based on viewing the learner as an active participant who processes information cognitively, emotionally and through practice, individually and in interaction with the environment or with others, in order to create understanding, manageability, skills and meaningfulness. Effective learning integrates theoretical understanding with opportunities to practise concrete strategies. Approaches to learning are equally applicable to patient learning as to learning in education. These include creating a positive learning environment and dialogue, supporting memory and meaningful learning, enabling diverse ways of learning, and providing opportunities for practice, reflection and feedback. These approaches can help participants feel confident in trying new strategies, receiving feedback, and gradually integrating new skills into their daily work.

Developing Salutogenic Competence

Based on the *Think and Act Patient Learning* framework, applying a salutogenic approach does not necessarily require additional resources; rather, it may reduce resource demands because the resulting benefits promote health and well-being. Working within an organisational context shaped by policy, productivity demands and efficiency expectations, without compromising safety or patient and staff satisfaction, can often feel difficult to influence. The following example illustrates how a salutogenic perspective, including the concept of SOC, can provide a foundation for a person-centred organisation focused on patient learning. Central to this is ensuring that both healthcare staff and patients feel involved in decision-making and that care is comprehensible, manageable and meaningful.

A unit within a nursing home for patients with dementia was at risk of closure because of complaints from relatives who were dissatisfied with the care provided, particularly inadequate hygiene routines and lack of outdoor visits. Municipal officials responsible for elderly care decided to investigate the underlying causes of the conflict. They chose to apply a salutogenic perspective at the nursing home, focusing on healthy and supportive factors rather than only on problems affecting staff and patients. A series of workshops designed to identify these factors was conducted by external specialists, separately with unit managers and staff.

During these workshops, it became clear that managers and staff shared several strengths, including a strong value base and a positive work climate characterised by humour, joy, mutual appreciation and flexibility. Staff expressed pride in their work and strong commitment to patients. They also described how they created a homelike atmosphere, for example, by baking every day, and emphasised their trust in leadership. At the same time, they described tensions between established care routines and patients' individual wishes, such as not wanting to shower or go outdoors. Subsequent workshops focused on strengthening healthy and supportive factors based on the SOC components of comprehensibility, manageability and meaningfulness. To enhance comprehensibility, participants identified a need for continuous staff education in dementia care, clearer channels of information and an open dialogue in which opinions are valued. To support manageability, recommendations included greater staff involvement in decision-making, forums for sharing experiences and continuous feedback. To strengthen meaningfulness, managers were encouraged to acknowledge staff motivation, commitment to patient care and need for continuous learning. In meetings with patients and relatives, emphasis was placed on open and honest communication to achieve shared understanding, on adapting activities, on setting attainable goals and on encouraging motivation in a positive spirit. Based on the identified health-promoting and supportive factors, management developed questionnaires to evaluate work satisfaction and patient or relative satisfaction annually, followed by workshops with all staff members to identify priority areas for further improvement.

This example illustrates the importance of promoting knowledge (comprehensibility), providing effective strategies for problem-solving (manageability) and encouraging motivation and support (meaningfulness), thereby enabling staff to sustain a long-term person-centred approach in their work. The case focuses on dementia care and shows how a salutogenic approach can be applied in a complex setting in which pedagogical encounters play an important role in daily work. Competence development initiated at the municipal level (macro) increased awareness of how management (meso) and staff (micro) at the unit could improve communication with patients and relatives to develop shared understanding. The example also highlights the importance of evaluation, a key aspect of person-centred care, in achieving long-term impact in implementation.

Developing Health Literacy Competence

Health literacy education aims to help participants understand its importance and develop the communication skills needed to support patients in navigating healthcare. It can be organised in different ways, from a single lecture to a longer course or workshop delivered over several sessions. Regardless of format, theory and practice should be closely integrated, with activities designed to promote active engagement. Such activities may include reflection, discussion and opportunities to practise concrete strategies, for example, avoiding medical jargon, rephrasing information, structuring explanations clearly, and using visual or written supports during patient encounters. Interactive approaches encourage participants to experiment, ask questions, and gain confidence in communication. Ideally, teaching takes place across several sessions, with progression that helps participants move from awareness and understanding to active consideration and application in clinical work. Repeated opportunities to revisit communication strategies deepen learning.

It is usually helpful to begin by explaining what health literacy is, why it matters, and how it can be supported in practice. Patient cases work well. Short films in which people with limited health literacy describe challenging healthcare situations can make the topic feel real and relevant. These stories bring patients' voices into the room, help participants recognise common challenges and often make the topic more engaging and meaningful. When introducing practical work with health literacy, it is useful to present a range of strategies that can be applied both organisationally and in individual patient encounters. Adult learners are often curious and want practical examples of what can be done in daily work beyond simply understanding the concept. Clear and concrete suggestions help participants see how health literacy can be translated into everyday communication strategies in daily work.

If time and resources allow, participants can explore different strategies through structured training activities. Active and practice-oriented methods are particularly valuable for skill development. Examples of activities include:

- Participants brainstorm and write down medical jargon and abbreviations that patients may find difficult to understand. They then develop simpler alternatives and share them with the group for feedback.

- Participants work in pairs using pictorial support, for example, communication boards with multiple images, and practise speaking while pointing to the pictures. One person acts as the healthcare provider and the other as the patient. Participants can also search for or create pictorial materials tailored to specific patient groups. Afterwards, they discuss how the communication felt, what worked well and what could be improved.
- Participants practise the teach-back method in pairs or groups of three. One person acts as the provider, one as the patient and a third may observe. The provider receives a short text, for example, on healthy eating, physical activity, a diagnosis or medicine use, and uses it as the basis for a conversation. The focus is on clear communication through selecting key information, limiting content, using plain language and educational materials, and asking the patient to explain the information in their own words. Afterwards, participants discuss what worked well and what could be improved from a health literacy perspective.

During training, participants need to feel safe. This can be supported by using small groups, avoiding role-play in front of the whole class, and making several rooms available. It is also helpful to emphasise that learners are encouraged to experiment and reflect in order to find communication approaches that work for them and for the patients they meet, and that there is rarely only one correct approach.

Another important part of health literacy education is exploring how health-literacy supportive practices appear in real clinical environments. This may involve observing communication in patient encounters, analysing written or digital patient materials from the perspective of different patient groups, or using checklists to access whether health literacy principles are applied. Such activities allow participants to reflect on how communication takes place, how information is conveyed and how easy or difficult the organisation is for patients to navigate. These observations provide insight into patient safety, equity and person-centred care. Linking health literacy to core professional competences reinforces its relevance.

Guiding learners through observation and reflection on how health-literacy supportive practices and structures appear in different healthcare settings can be challenging. Learners may become frustrated when they notice shortcomings but feel unable to influence them. One way to address this is to link these experiences to organisational health literacy by emphasising that improvement must occur at multiple levels of the healthcare system. While participants cannot be expected to change everything, everyday communication practices and professional choices can still make a meaningful difference to the patients they meet.

After classroom-based practice and observation, participants can apply one or more health-literacy supportive methods in real clinical settings, either in the workplace or during clinical placement. They should then reflect on these experiences with supervisors or peers. Engaging in a cycle of observing, testing and reflecting helps participants understand how communication approaches function with different patients and under different conditions. Reflection on what worked well, what was challenging and what might be adjusted strengthens future application in clinical encounters. However, opportunities to practise and discuss experiences may vary depending on clinical supervisors, patient cases and local communication culture. Low awareness of health literacy in the clinical environment may lead to supportive practices being questioned or may limit constructive feedback. One way to reduce this challenge is to ensure that all staff in the clinical environment, or at least designated supervisors, receive an introduction to health literacy and clear information about the learner's task of practising and reflecting on different strategies. Even brief discussions of what worked well, what felt challenging and why can strengthen learning and encourage continued development. Such reflection also helps learners understand how context and communication culture shape what is possible in practice and supports the integration of health literacy skills into professional identity. In staff training, managers also need to be involved and understand the purpose so that staff can apply what has been learnt.

An alternative or complement to onsite training is digital and flexible learning, which can increase accessibility and allow learners to engage with content at their own pace. Online modules, recorded lectures and interactive quizzes make it possible to revisit key ideas when needed, which is especially useful when clinical schedules limit opportunities for group teaching. To ensure accessibility for diverse learners, it is helpful to offer information in multiple formats, for example, text, images, transcripts, or subtitles. Providing information in several modes supports learners with different linguistic, cultural and educational backgrounds and aligns with the principles of Universal Design for Learning, an approach that emphasises accessible teaching for diverse groups of learners (Kotcherlakota et al., 2024). However, not all healthcare professionals have access to their own computer, and finding time to complete training can be difficult. It is therefore helpful if online learning is also accessible by mobile phone and, where possible, scheduled into the working day.

Informal course evaluations and spontaneous feedback from participants in health literacy education, including both students and healthcare professionals, consistently indicate that structured, practice-oriented health literacy education is well received and perceived as useful. Learners often report gaining new insights and feeling motivated to try new communication strategies in clinical work. At the same time, practical conditions, such as time pressure or established ways of working in a clinical setting, may affect both opportunities to participate in training and the ease with which new approaches can be put into practice.

Developing Pedagogical Competence

During professional education, healthcare students learn what future practice requires in theory and practical skills, but they receive much less training in understanding learning itself, whether their own learning processes or those of the patients they will support. As part of a specialist nursing programme in cancer care, a new course design was introduced to increase participants' awareness of what learning can mean for patients and to strengthen their own pedagogical competence (Engqvist Boman et al., 2022). The learning activities required participants to:

- Reflect on their own previous learning experiences in order to become aware of their pre-understanding.
- Study and discuss learning theories with peers to deepen understanding of learning processes.
- Read about and discuss the concept of the pedagogical encounter in seminars with teachers.
- Identify and observe pedagogical encounters in clinical cancer care and apply understanding of learning to patients' situations.
- Articulate observations, experiences and reflections on patients' learning as well as their own, in written assignments and discussions with peers and teachers.
- Plan and conduct a pedagogical encounter with a patient, observed by a "critical friend," either a peer or a clinical supervisor, who provided constructive feedback on performance.
- Act as a critical friend by observing and giving feedback to a peer, colleague or clinical supervisor.
- Write a description of the pedagogical encounter, emphasising personal learning and grounding the reasoning in learning theories, both generally and in relation to patients' learning and understanding.
- Organise and carry out an interprofessional seminar on patient learning in the clinical setting, focusing on the participant's ability to facilitate healthcare staff learning about patient learning.

Participants' perceptions of the course and their performance in written assignments were evaluated. The most appreciated activities were studying learning theories, observing a pedagogical encounter, acting as a critical friend and documenting personal pedagogical encounters. Less appreciated were conducting a pedagogical encounter personally and having a critical friend. The main reason was clinical supervisors' limited knowledge of pedagogical encounters and how to provide feedback on student performance. Although this activity was not highly valued in the questionnaire, students demonstrated both ability and appreciation in performing and analysing their pedagogical encounter in their written assignments. Feeling safe, trusting the critical friend, receiving feedback and having both strengths and areas for improvement acknowledged were all important for learning.

In written assignments based on observations of others' pedagogical encounters in the clinic, participants reflected on nurses' and physicians' behaviour, what was said, the interactions among all actors in the encounter, and patients' reactions. They mainly described and reflected on patients' learning, with limited attention to their own. When writing about pedagogical encounters they had conducted themselves, most participants demonstrated well-planned activities, including clear descriptions and discussions aligned with the structure of the learning situations. They reflected not only on their own learning but also on the patient's situation and the conditions that supported learning. A basic factor was establishing dialogue in a safe environment by starting from patients' questions, pre-understanding, perceptions and needs. Participants' reflections and reasoning were grounded in relevant literature, indicating increased awareness and understanding of learning processes. These results were confirmed in interviews with a selected group of nurses who had participated in the course; they described how they thought and acted in pedagogical encounters with patients (Gustavell et al., 2025). They described a holistic perspective on patients' situations, with the overall goal of supporting understanding and management of illness. Important factors included creating an atmosphere of trust, striving for mutual understanding and facilitating patient participation. Their thoughts and actions in encounters with patients were supported by what had been experienced and studied about learning in the course, by nursing competences and above all by personal characteristics and experiences. Overall, the evaluation showed that participants increased awareness of their pedagogical role and of thinking and acting patient learning (Engqvist Boman et al., 2022). However, more time was needed to discuss and process learning theories in order to strengthen understanding and use of them. Participants also found that nurses in the clinic had limited pedagogical knowledge and were therefore unable to provide feedback on performance during the pedagogical encounter. Although healthcare organisations and universities collaborate closely, universities lack the authority to determine the development of pedagogical skills among healthcare professionals. To further develop the course and improve opportunities for feedback, participants were encouraged to present and discuss the model for pedagogical encounters with clinical supervisors, thereby contributing to shared understanding of its meaning. The course was continuously revised in line with evaluations and assessments from previous cohorts. This contributed to increased participant satisfaction with the learning activities and to greater awareness of how to support patient learning.

Reflecting on this example, certain contextual factors at macro, meso and micro levels help explain their influence on the development, implementation and sustainability of the course. At the macro level in Sweden, university teachers are required to demonstrate pedagogical competence as a condition of employment, in accordance with the Swedish Higher Education Ordinance and recommendations from the Association of Swedish Higher Education Institutions. At the meso level, the medical university offering the specialist nursing programme is required to engage in continuous pedagogical competence development for teachers and students. Pedagogical development serves as a quality indicator that is followed up annually in each department and unit. The course was developed as an educational research project funded by the regional council and the university. At the micro level, the course was grounded in learning theories, and participants were encouraged to study, experience, and apply knowledge continuously in ways that supported their learning. Although no evaluation of the interaction among these levels has been conducted, it is reasonable to assume that requirements for pedagogical competence within medicine and healthcare education support implementation of this form of competence development.

Summary

Successful implementation of developmental work such as the *Think and Act Patient Learning* framework is a challenging and complex process. It depends on contextual factors at macro, meso and micro levels and is facilitated by dynamic interaction among them. A value-based organisational culture grounded in salutogenic and person-centred care is an important prerequisite for implementation. Practical structures and support at all levels are also essential. Patient learning is an individual and dynamic process that must permeate healthcare professionals' pedagogical encounters, with the goal of promoting health and well-being. Developing health literacy competence is a key part of this work, shaping how communication, information and learning are supported in everyday practice. The commitment and competence of individual caregivers are essential, but sustainable results also require a healthcare system that supports these efforts. This chapter has also highlighted the importance of the rapid digitalisation of healthcare and of societal organisations that support patients in self-care management. Through these developments, patients will increasingly develop knowledge about their own health, which will then be brought into pedagogical encounters and should be recognised and valued by healthcare professionals.

References

Bate, P. (2014). Context is everything. In *Perspectives on context.* The Health Foundation, 90 Long Acre, London WC2E 9RA. ISBN 978-1-906461-51-5

Boman, E. L., Sandelin, K., Wengström, Y., & Silén, C. (2018). Patients' participation during treatment and care of breast cancer—A possibility and an imperative. *European Journal of Oncology Nursing*, 37, 35–42. https://doi.org/10.1016/j.ejon.2018.09.002.

Brach, C., Keller, D., Hernandez, L. M., Baur, C., Parker, R., Dreyer, B., Schyve, P., Lemerise, A. J., & Schillinger, D. (2012). *Ten attributes of health literate health care organizations*. Institute of Medicine. https://nam.edu/wpcontent/uploads/2015/06/BPH_Ten_HLit_Attributes.pd

Centers for Disease Control and Prevention. (2023). *What is health literacy?* https://www.cdc.gov/healthliteracy/learn/index.html

Doble, E., Robson, A., Kar, P., & Reidy, C. (2024). Peer support in chronic health conditions. *BMJ*, 386, e070443. https://doi.org/10.1136/bmj-2022-070443

Ehk, S., Petersson, S., Khalaf, A., & Nilsson, M. (2024). Nurses' experiences of integrating the salutogenic perspective with person-centered care for older people in Swedish nursing home care: An interview-based qualitative study. *BMC Geriatrics*, 24(1), 262. https://doi.org/10.1186/s12877-024-04831-7

Ekman, I., Ebrahimi, Z., & Olaya Contreras, P. (2021). Person-centred care: Looking back, looking forward. *European Journal of Cardiovascular Nursing*, 20(2), 93–95. https://doi.org/10.1093/eurjcn/zvaa025

Elliott, M. J., Love, S., Fox, D. E., Verdin, N., Donald, M., Manns, K., Cunningham, D., Goth, J., & Hemmelgarn, B. R. (2022). 'It's the empathy'-defining a role for peer support among people living with chronic kidney disease: A qualitative study. *BMJ Open*, 12(5), e057518. https://doi.org/10.1136/bmjopen-2021-057518

Engqvist Boman, L., Sundberg, K., Petersson, L. M., Backman, M., & Silén, C. (2022). A pedagogical model to enhance nurses' ability to support patient learning: An educational design research study. *International Journal of Medical Education*, 13, 176–186. https://doi.org/10.5116/ijme.62c2.b9c4

Farmanova, E., Bonneville, L., & Bouchard, L. (2018). Organizational health literacy: Review of theories, frameworks, guides, and implementation issues. *Inquiry: The Journal of Health Care Organization, Provision, and Financing*, 55, 1–17. https://doi.org/10.1177/0046958018757848

Førland, G. (2014). *Learning in health: Educational foundation and practice of the Learning and Mastery Centre* (Doctoral dissertation, Karolinska Institutet). https://hdl.handle.net/10616/42

Fulop, N., & Robert, G. (2015). *Context for successful quality improvement.* The Health Foundation.

Gustavell, T., Silén, C., Petersson, L. M., & Boman, L. E. (2025). How experienced nurses think and act in supporting patient learning: An interview study. *BMC Nursing*, 24, 869. https://doi.org/10.1186/s12912-025-03542-7

Hang, L., Zhang, J., Lu, Z., Xu, J., & Chen, Y. (2024). Effectiveness of ePRO-based symptom management for cancer patients: A systematic review and meta-analysis of randomized controlled studies. *Supportive Care in Cancer*, 32(12), 842. https://doi.org/10.1007/s00520-024-09026-9

Keeling, A., Downey, J., Halkes, M., & Wei, Y. (2025). The impact of patient-generated health data from mobile health technologies on health care management and clinical decision-making: Narrative scoping review. *Journal of Medical Internet Research*, 27, e77359. https://doi.org/10.2196/77359

Kotcherlakota, S., Stamler, L. L., Clark, A., & Howell, M. C. (2024). Implementing universal design for learning in nursing education: Faculty perspectives. *Teaching and Learning in Nursing*, 19(1), e138–e144. https://doi.org/10.1016/j.teln.2023.10.0031

Langius-Eklöf, A., Crafoord, M. T., Christiansen, M., Fjell, M., & Sundberg, K. (2017). Effects of an interactive mHealth innovation for early detection of patient-reported symptom distress with focus on participatory care: Protocol for a study based on prospective, randomized, controlled trials in patients with prostate and breast cancer. *BMC Cancer*, 17(1), 466. https://doi.org/10.1186/s12885-017-3450-y

Langius-Eklöf, A., Craftman, Å. G., Gellerstedt, L., Kelmendi, N., Rooth, K., Gustavell, T., & Sundberg, K. (2025). Digital and nurse-led support intervention in primary care during the first year after curative intent treatment for breast or prostate cancer: Study protocol of two cluster randomised controlled pilot trials. *BMJ Open*, 15(2), e090848. https://doi.org/10.1136/bmjopen-2024-090848

Madanian, S., Nakarada-Kordic, I., Reay, S., & Chetty, T. (2023). Patients' perspectives on digital health tools. *PEC Innovation*, 2, 100171. https://doi.org/10.1016/j.pecinn.2023.100171

McCormack, B., McCane, T., Bulley, K., Brown, D., McMillan, A., & Martin, S. (2021). *Fundamentals of person-centered healthcare practice*. John Wiley and Sons Ltd.

M-POHL. (2023). *Health literacy policies – How can they be developed and implemented? A guide for policy and decision makers*. International Coordination Center of M-POHL at the Austrian National Public Health Institute. https://m-pohl.net/sites/m-pohl.net/files/2024-03/Guide_health-literacy-policies.pdf

Ocloo, J., Goodrich, J., Tanaka, H., Birchall-Searle, J., Dawson, D., & Farr, M. (2020). The importance of power, context and agency in improving patient experience through a patient and family centred care approach. *Health Research Policy and Systems*, 18(1), 10. https://doi.org/10.1186/s12961-019-0487-1

Palant, A., & Himmel, W. (2019). Are there also negative effects of social support? A qualitative study of patients with inflammatory bowel disease. *BMJ Open*, 9(1), e022642. https://doi.org/10.1136/bmjopen-2018-022642

Smith, F., Hellström, A., Gunnarsdóttir, K. Á., Genell, A., Eriksson, E., Mannefred, C., Björk-Eriksson, T., & Vaughn, L. (2021). Exploring the meaning, role and experiences of a patient-led social innovation for people affected by cancer: A new collaborative care model complementing traditional cancer rehabilitation in Sweden. *BMJ Open Quality*, 10(4), e001400. https://doi.org/10.1136/bmjoq-2021-001400

Sørensen, K., Levin-Zamir, D., Duong, T. V., Okan, O., Brasil, V. V., & Nutbeam, D. (2021). Building health literacy system capacity: A framework for health literate systems. *Health Promotion International*, 36(Suppl. 1), i13–i23. https://doi.org/10.1093/heapro/daab153

World Health Organization. (2021). *Global strategy on digital health 2020–2025*. https://www.who.int/publications/i/item/9789240020924

World Health Organization Regional Office for Europe. (2022). *Equity within digital health technology within the WHO European Region: A scoping review*. https://www.who.int/europe/publications/i/item/WHO-EURO-2022-6810-46576-67595

World Health Organization Regional Office for Europe. (2023). *Therapeutic patient education: An introductory guide*. https://apps.who.int/iris/handle/10665/371286

INDEX

Note: Numbers in **bold** indicate a table. Numbers in *italics* indicate a figure. Numbers that are <u>underlined</u> indicate a box.

For Product Safety Concerns and Information please contact our EU representative GPSR@taylorandfrancis.com
Taylor & Francis Verlag GmbH, Kaufingerstraße 24, 80331 München, Germany

www.ingramcontent.com/pod-product-compliance
Ingram Content Group UK Ltd.
Pitfield, Milton Keynes, MK11 3LW, UK
UKHW021909281026
477140UK00011B/395
* 9 7 8 1 0 3 2 8 9 0 2 5 8 *